I0455156

CHRONIC PAIN.

HAND IN HAND

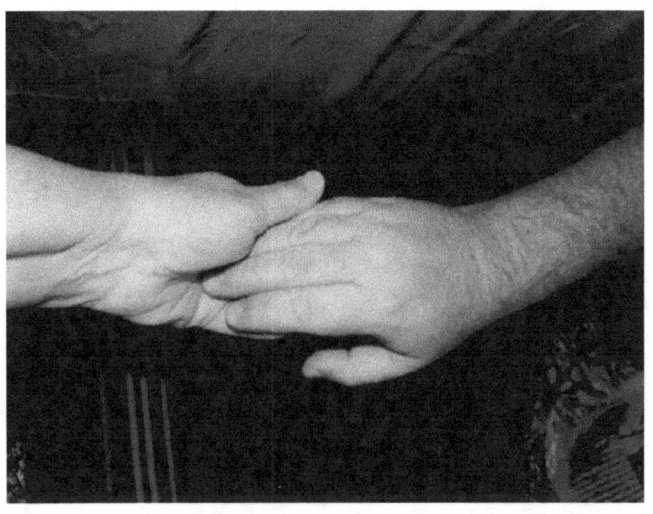

Ideas to Make Living With Chronic Pain Easier

BY

Sherry E. Showalter
PhD, LCSW, BCD, M.Msc

AND

John Argent
Full Time Caretaker

Copyright ©2012 Sherry E. Showalter & John Argent
All rights reserved
ISBN-10: 1478304596
ISBN-13: 978-1478304593

INTRODUCTION

This is a book about chronic pain. Hand in hand; two people sharing the thoughts and ways to help walking in pain easier. It is a book to assist those who suffer; those who live day to day with chronic pain and the discoveries that come from those encounters between being one in pain and one who has professionally and personally provided care and time.

We know you very well for we are you. We know you perhaps as well as anybody in the world for we have listened to your stories with patience and attention and we have been greatly rewarded and humbled by each step and each hand we have touched.

We have been touched with the deep recesses of your thoughts and fears and the memories of the appalling experiences that are so often the origin of chronic pain. We offer no treatments here; only thoughts and ideas to share, through stories and alternatives to compliment what you may already have in place.

We have been honored, we have been saddened and yet we are blessed and often we have been bold and imaginative. Our wish is that you gain greater understanding of the kaleidoscopes of healing ways to best benefit you and enhance life with those you love along the path into wellness.

Our hope and intention for this book is to offer some suggestions that may provide some more relief and enhance what your physician may prescribe for you and to help you build some emotional tools to use in dealing with chronic pain.

Please check with a doctor before trying any of these methods. These methods are not intended to replace what your doctor does, but rather to enhance what your doctor is doing for your chronic pain.

The mind is a wonderful tool if we open our senses and allow the many facets of the mind to work. We hope you find that these methods help make your life a little better.

PART ONE

CHRONIC PAIN IN ITS MANY DIMENSIONS

BY

Dr. Sherry E. Showalter

Chronic Pain

Pain is a word that is often associated with an unpleasant sensory and/or emotional experience more often associated with actual or potential bone or tissue damage or described in terms of such damage in a medical model of care. It is a word that has been associated with health and wellness, and attended to by a medical model of care, but it is also a word/feeling that is applied to emotional/spiritual sensory experiences as well.

Pain is subjective, therefore treatment of pain is complex and unquestionably an unpleasant experience for the one experiencing it and those who love them to witness. Pain is difficult to treat, even now with us knowing so much more than ever before.

Pain has been described as a feeling of distress, suffering or agony. It is often physical in nature and is caused by stimulation of nerve endings with the neurotransmitters sending messages from the brain center, with the purpose being to protect, warn, or indicate that something is wrong.

Chronic would indicate on-going, unrelenting pain; rather like an unwelcomed guest at a picnic such as an ant bite, that just irritates or stays with you. It is sometimes a nuisance, and at other times becomes larger than life, and has the sting of a wasp's nest that fell from nowhere covering you on a beautiful day without warning; and its effects are felt long after a joyous moment has been experienced. Those who state they have "chronic" conditions are never far from their conditions and try to stay close to home, to bathrooms, to medicines if available in order to be prepared.

We've all heard the words "chronic worry" and "chronic bronchitis". Many medical dictionaries will assist one in clarifying "chronic pain" with the following definition: Pain that continues or recurs over a prolonged period, caused by various diseases or abnormal conditions in the body, a part of the body, and affects the nervous system, immune system. It can be less intense than acute pain, but often a constant in someone's life.

The person who suffers chronic pain does not always have increased pulse and rapid respirations as those are autonomic reactions to pain that cannot be sustained for long periods. The chronic pain sufferer has re-set that part of the brain.

Chronic pain sufferers are complex to treat as their conditions make pain management programs difficult secondary to the varied diagnosis and conditions that they may have. All becomes a delicate balancing act requiring specialists in the field of pain management and skillful interventionists.

More than 80% of all physician visits are for chronic pain, and yet the majority of health care providers have little or no training specific to pain medicine or pain management! We now can read statistics that let us know that an estimated $100 billion is spent annually in medical claims, disability payments and lost productivity. And yes, that does include those fraudulent claims as well. There are those who still bilk a system with feigned complaints and illnesses while others who need services are denied.

We are starting to see the medical communities realize the tremendous importance of moving from a strict medical model to one that is more holistic in its approach to a patient centered focus of care. We must employ alternative healing modalities to address the many layers of complex patient needs who suffer from chronic pain to address the physical/spiritual/emotional facets of pain, while empowering patients to employ all that is within them as they struggle to break through their pain.

The stakes are now at an all-time high for prescription drug use and abuse: physicians are having to decipher who is in need of management of illness vs. those who are looking to abuse a system for personal gain or misuse of prescription drugs making those with chronic pain having to seek pain specialists and travel greater distances the reality for many.

This is a delicate balance and one that the world is finding to be a great challenge in monitoring and accessing. Advocacy is needed for those in precarious health to be sure they have access to needed services and to enhance their care and abilities to live life with less pain and a plan of care that is managed with a pain regiment closely monitored and adhered to alone with complimentary therapies that have been documented to assist in pain relief while enhancing quality of life for those who suffer with chronic pain.

The brain has a remarkable ability to assist in healing pathways through endorphins and the inhibition of pain transmission by tactile signals that have yet to be fully tapped with techniques of relaxations, massage, applications that utilize sensory motor enhancements to pain medications and traditional medicine approaches. Medical communities are just beginning to embrace these modalities of care.

We see pain assessment tools and pain scales that through time patients have not understood fully, and in their attempts to be taken seriously they have indicated pain on the highest of a pain scale, only then to be not taken seriously when asked where their pain lies. Through education and continued re-assessment can we empower patients in understanding of those scales while truly paying attention in attending to their needs and their very real perceptions of their pain.

Objective signs of pain and subjective reports of pain have longstanding histories of being very differently reported. During the last several years we have observed patients who appear in pain clinics and in ER's drug seeking in the guise of pain suffering, thereby making the medical community on higher alert and ultimately those who are chronic, ill and in pain are the ones paying the highest price and living in pain without proper medications.

The psycho-social-spiritual aspects of chronic pain are numerous, and have yet to be discussed fully in professional or personal blogs or journals. The tolerance of pain and a person's reactions to pain become less easy to identify and more complex than physiologic responses that are measurable it seems.

An individuals' response to pain is subject to so many influences including their body, beliefs, culture, faith, spirituality, religion. They include their previous experiences with pain, what they are led to believe they can deal with, live with, suffer with; how they respond to pain and discomfort, their state of well-being. How one copes with pain and their over-all feelings and fatigue determine their abilities to function not only daily but also on an hour to hour basis.

A person in pain is often seen grimacing, having difficulty concentrating or remembering. And there are times one who is ill or filled with pain, may present to you as rather self-absorbed as they are now pre-occupied with pain/illness, and the myriad of changes that are happening in their bodies and they are unable to deal with the world around them.

Chronic pain is life altering. Those with chronic pain grieve losses daily, as they find they can no longer do as they once did, their lives take a path that is unfamiliar and many feel out of balance and afraid. It can be life stopping, life altering, and yet, it can be an opportunity for deep understanding and great growth when employing all the senses and means of understanding along with the tools that are readily available to heal from within.

Pain control has come a long way through the years, with specialists now becoming attuned to the individual experiencing chronic pain and the vivid kaleidoscope of colors of pain along with the connection to the neurotransmitters of the brain. People are being taught to re-wire their brains and to utilize the sensory motor skills to re-work pain pathways, along with complimentary medicines and healing modalities to relieve pain.

Research has demonstrated that neuronal circuitry and internal systems are also linked to faith and hope allows one to assist in decreasing pain in the body, the mind, the spirit and soul. Signals arising from stimulation of neurons in the gray matter of the brain stem travel downward to the dorsal horns of the spinal cord where incoming pain impulses from the periphery terminate! It is complex, considering we still do not fully understand the wonderment of our brain, but we do now understand that it is so very complex and yet we control more than we ever realized.

So it stands to reason, that we can control much of our thoughts about life, death, dying and in addition PAIN. We now are aware of the benefit of "distraction techniques" as some would call it. Many prefer to call it "self-soothing", or "alternative healing".

Massage/gentle pressure can be particularly effective during high pain crisis for many. That feel can activate the thick-fiber impulses and produce a preponderance of tactile signals that compete with pain signals in the brain and body. Massage is "touch", and touch is healing by its very nature.

Gentle touch to many is a signal of love during times of pain, or high stress, or heartache, indicating that one is cared for and about. Touch also can improve circulations in the body, assist in re-positioning the body and limbs gently and promote muscle relaxation that will allow the relief of spasms, pain signals, and angst secondary to both the pain signals and spasms.

There are specific relaxation techniques that can be taught; can be thought up by those suffering chronic pain, that can aide, relieve, reduce physical and mental tension and stress, thereby reducing pain. These techniques have been used on infants, children, teens, adults and elders for centuries, in hospices around the world, and typically begin with a soothing voice or touch.

Many have said they "do not believe", or "it is hard to learn these things", but once the time is taken to explore alternatives to healing and to practice them one can achieve mastery. At first it is difficult to focus; there is fear of only adding to the pain for those who are suffering pain. Like anything new; there is resistance at first! As with anything it seems once a person is open to receiving, the benefits outweigh the fear or cost, and the benefits have been well documented as worth the time and trouble in the management of chronic and ongoing pain.

Many through the years are advocates of using heat/cold when symptoms flare; again these are additions to a well thought out and implemented pain management program for the chronic pain sufferer. It is as different as each fingerprint on what is effective and for whom; along with liniments, ointments, salves and balms.

Some will swear by tiger balm, while others make a home remedy of ole timey herbs; and still others will sleep with a sharp knife under the bed in order to and believe that it will "cut the pain". One thing is certain; those who suffer chronic pain are challenged to find ways to enrich their lives in order to live the best they can.

The International Association for the Study of Pain has denoted that pain which is persistent, often lasting more than six months and has symptoms that may be the same as indicated for acute pain is classified as "chronic pain". What was once thought to "be all in your head", has been studied, researched, and continues to leave many baffled even today, while many pray for relief and are a part of a Universal energy Circle or prayer group.

Cancer pain is one of the three categories that are studied along with acute pain, and chronic pain. Palliative medicine has some of the brightest of the bright in pain management in the worlds now; that are the real experts in treating pain and incorporate alternative methods of employing non-traditional modalities in their efforts of relieving pain.

There is also a classification known as "pain disorder" also known as a "somatoform" disorder, which is hard to control and is related to psychological conflicts made worse by environmental stressors. It is a horrible pain; one best treated through psychotherapy once medical conditions are ruled out to be the root cause.

Chronic pain takes a tremendous toll on a person; on the workplace, on the families as people attempt to make adjustments to their schedules. Often having increased absenteeism from work, many having to see multiple doctors at various times, or are frequent visitors to ER's around the country when pain is out of control.

With chronic pain, one will notice that many people withdraw from activities, begin to stay close to home, for fear of an exacerbation of pain. Often accompanying this pain is disease and body breakdown along with issues of loss/grief.

Families become increasingly tired of hearing and feeling helpless, which adds to the real and physical pain and limited mobility by those who are now also weakened in their immune systems, and also feeling guilt secondary to needing extra help from others.

Those who have been used to independence now find they may be unable to participate in things as they once did. They now find that they are no longer able to work, may begin the arduous journey of filing for disability, have increased physician visits, decreased incomes, and justifications of illness, increased stress and decreased feelings of self-esteem and self-worth.

The complications and complexities again are like a kaleidoscope that is out of focus and often lost its brilliance clouded by fear, uncertainty and a life filled with pain that is not well attended to. It becomes increasingly vital for those suffering chronic pain along with the friends and families to learn ways to empower and assist in mastering alternative healing modalities that will aide, relieve and alleviate pain when possible in order to enhance the quality of life for those who are living with pain in our world.

Awareness and education are the beginning steps toward a path of addressing the issues at hand of "chronic pain" for those enduring those sleepless days and nights. It is in awareness and education for people, families and friends that light can penetrate the darkness while addressing chronic pain, the diminished feelings of self-worth and increase a person's quality of life.

Speaking to thousands of people one thing is certain; from little ones to Elders, all will tell you, "I can handle just about anything, if people will tell me just what it is I am facing." With that being said, people do much better when they understand their illness, condition; their medications and their abilities' to self-regulate, to divert their attention and to send signals to the brain/body/spirit and to choose to be more than their illness, disease or their pain. When one who lives with chronic pain feels they are losing control by inches, day in and day out, it can be overwhelming.

How a person "chooses" to live with that is in fact a choice that is made each day by millions of people living with disease and pain. As one woman explained it "I wake each day in horrible pain, yet I choose to smile. It is a choice that is still mine to make." That is a profound statement and speaks loudly to the resilience of the human spirit in pain or not in pain. Many things are within our control and there are choices we make no matter if we are well, ill, able or disabled. And these choices can and do affect how we move into the day just as alternative therapies can and do enhance our management of pain in its many dimensions, in loss, grief, and healing.

Attitude remains a key ingredient to how people cope and more from surviving to thriving as I was taught by a beautiful woman who was a walking testament to that reality and lives in chronic and horrific pain. We as people need to be validated, to be honored in our journey, in our happiness, our struggles, our pain, our losses and our grief. We need to be assisted along the way, and perhaps by lending a hand, an ear or at times a suggestion is the best we have to give; if given authentically to another.

It is hard to imagine walking in the shoes of one who walks each day in horrific pain. Imagine if you will for a moment: you have just walked up to a socket, knowing full well the effects of sticking your finger in that socket. You then place your finger in there and you do not remove it, but the shock goes through your body and YOU FEEEL IT. It just keeps going long after you remove your finger, it continues.

For many, that is their chronic pain; it is reported as that very feeling; someone just puts a finger or their whole body in a socket that takes them from a smiling and otherwise fine day; and then it happens; a body is seized in that pain... and it just lasts. At some point it is not so strong, but the effects linger, the exhaustion secondary to it profound, rendering them weak, tired, unsettled, confused by it, fearful of the next time... that is chronic and remarkable PAIN.

Then, if you will, imagine trying to describe that to a friend or loved one and hearing "I've been feeling the same way!", or hearing "Oh, my Aunt Jane had that. Just take a nap and you will get over it and be fine in no time!". That is the most disparaging support that a person in chronic pain will ever hear.

Think about it, would you feel supported and loved or would you feel that your pain was being diminished by their comments? People are just not comfortable hearing of another person's suffering, pain, loss, or grief. They open their mouths, the tongue falls out and people immediately step on it or in it....

Yet, a person with a positive outlook, one who looks at the outlet as a mountain and declares, "I see you, now get out of my way!" That chronic pain sufferer is a person who learns and masters all modalities in order to live as independently as possible, to know they are not their disease; they have to fight in order to get through their days. They become their best advocate in medical communities, search the internet and read the latest on alternative healing routes, listen to suggestions and filter out what may or may not be beneficial to them.

People who choose this path understand that there will be days that are manageable and that sometimes the adrenalin surge of great excitement or pleasurable visits, or experiences will fuel them, and they will self-manage their conditions in order to achieve maximum functions for the best quality of life they can have.

Will there be concessions? Will there be times when they pay dearly for having a great time, or for going to great lengths to do things that regular people take for granted (i.e. a ride in a car, sitting too long enjoying the company of another at the kitchen table, dinner with friends)?

Absolutely, once the adrenalin runs out, the medicines are late in the taking; the body says you have over extended our sitting up time today or last night. But, one who enjoys their brief time on this earth will not give in or give up secondary to limitations, but will live life fully and will utilize each and every ideal presented to enhance their ability to self-regulate and decrease pain and suffering if they choose to.

We are limited in our abilities by our imaginations; disease, pain, and loss will limit at times the ability, but never the mind or strength of choice. Many who suffer chronic pain are so caught up in the physiological aspects of the pain that they cannot see the impact it has on everyone they love. At times they are unable to help that at the time; but when the realization is discovered one will often hear the stories of their remorse, their sadness that life has affected so many that are loved so dearly.

Chronic pain and disease can be all consuming, affecting actions, motivation, and much of a person's thoughts. Fears of "what is next" or "waiting for the next shoe to drop, or the next pain/diagnosis" can rob many of the moments that are now. It is a normal and natural response to pain, exhaustion and loss.

The importance of treating chronic pain has never been stronger than today, as more and more people including children suffer chronic pain. Medications are not always the answer, as many have adverse reactions to medications; physicians are hesitant to increase the medications or to monitor closely and to attend to the myriad of needs and symptoms of patients with multiple health issues and pain needs.

Medication related problems these days would rank fifth among the leading causes of death in the United States if they were in themselves considered a disease. While opioids /analgesics/NSAIDS/ pain medications are a useful tool in the treatment of pain, there is currently such misuse that many in need of this medication are suffering secondary to that abuse in the country, while many around the globe are unable to get the needed medications at all.

Many pain sufferers report they are not being listened to by their providers, yet they cannot afford to see and be treated by a specialized pain management physician. It is and has been a vicious cycle that continues like a hurricane through the lives of millions. Yet few will embrace safe methods that are within them to ease and relive pain in very real and tangible ways. It may be that they are unaware or suspicious or that they are just weary secondary to pain.

Many have tried OTC's (over the counter medicines), are devoted to vitamins and minerals; still millions report chronic pain has changed their lives and not in a way that is good. Chronic pain is difficult to understand for the one experiencing it; and even more complex for those who love or care deeply for one yet not suffering the immediate pain themselves.

We witness those who find that pain exceeds their expectations in ways never imagined. It affects resiliency and intact coping mechanisms by inches; taking a toll on people and over time, thousands are able often with assistance to realize it has much to do with the many and continual losses that accompany a life filled with chronic pain.

Most will report that avenues to communication breaks down over time, understandings become misunderstandings; intimacy becomes distance while struggles take place of joined efforts in opportunities that are now viewed as tremendous challenges. Finances dwindle as resources are used for adaptations in homes and multiple doctor visits and specialty medications and treatments never tried before. There is no cure for chronic pain.

The challenges are multiplied when care giving becomes one of a full time job in addition to the job that must pay the bills, or a job is ended as a result of pain that becomes life altering. Many are left to face a world of uncertainty and others find friends and family disappear altogether, leaving them alone in a world of pain.

Yet there are those who say that friends step up, family move in to care for them; to empower them, and do not allow pain to be the central thread of a rich tapestry known to bond love and life that is much more than illness, disease and pain.

It would be wonderful if everyone had an advocate to accompany them to the many and painful visits to physicians often driven out of pain crisis, or new and disturbing findings from blood work, or CAT/MRI scans. There one hears reports of treatment received by office workers, nurses or aides that meet them with less than compassion only to be followed by a physician who then has little time to offer support and kindness.

It is through the eyes of a patient that one gets the perceptions that are reality for one who suffers greatly at the hands of a practitioner who has taken an oath to "Do No Harm" in a medical facility where harm can be done by the first minutes of a visit by the greeting or mannerisms in which a patient is treated.

Those who are trying to cope with pain, must also navigate cars, parking lots, elevators, and hallways just to arrive in uncomfortable seating, then wait until it is their turn. This typically heightens pain on a pain scale that is already above a 5 conservatively. Filling out paperwork, being greeted with anything less than kindness adds to distress for the person waiting to be seen. And then depending on the wait time, the mood of the physician and whether they have the previous records and memory intact, one never knows how the visit may go.

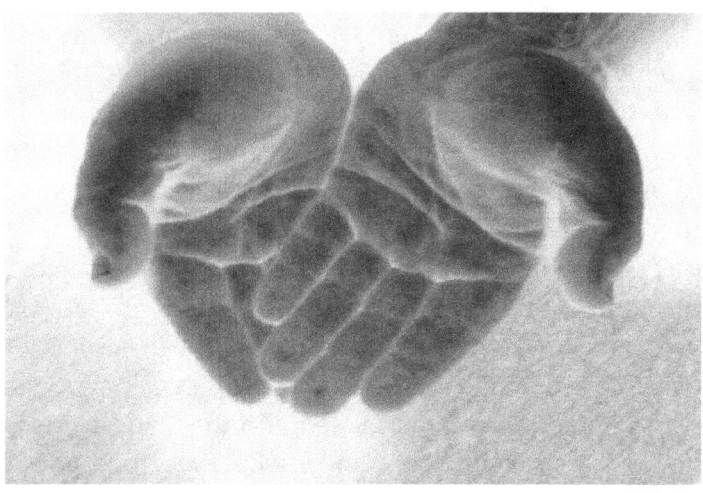

The patient if alone, has to navigate all of this, and hope that their pain will not block their ability to navigate the systems at play, nor play havoc on their memory or reasoning abilities while trying to comprehend all that is being said, and in addition saying all that they themselves need to say. It can be a daunting experience for one with a cold, and then add to that a person with a life limiting or chronic pain or disease ridden body, one can see how easy it is to feel powerless and out of control.

Loss of control for a person who suffers chronic pain is a large piece of the missing glass of the kaleidoscope of colors, just as a person diagnosed with a life threatening illness, it becomes the little but daily losses of independence that wear on a person over time.

The things that most would take for granted become enormous tasks that need to be accomplished or things that one must ask others for help in doing. The energy required to advocate for self is overwhelming at times, and can leave one feeling helpless when pain is out of control and those in power and positions of the helping professions are less than caring, compassionate and helpful. It adds to the pain, the burden, the decreased sense of self and heightens the sense of inability to move the pain. It can also prove deadly in terms of disease progression and a person's will to continue to fight.

The challenge becomes to enlist and maintain strong communication between health care providers, family and friends in order to be heard, to hear and to reach beyond the comfort zone in asking for what is needed; to re-state what may be obvious and to have a plan. A plan that is worked through, often at the expense of re-clarifying to people the need and the desire to be heard!

Physicians are people; they have their own time crunches, families and outside pressures; and they would do well to attend conferences, seminars to enhance their resiliency in order to continue to provide best practice for those that they serve. Patients can be their own best advocates by sending their doctors and nurses a letter after a visit to let them know what was good about the visit, what was and felt wrong, and ways to improve the communication for the next visit.

People do not know, what they do not know. We must be proactive to set the bar higher and to let folks know when something is good and when it is just wrong in our world, in order to receive treatment and care along the way that we are in need of.

Pain takes a tremendous amount of energy, leaving little left to deal with details and to re-hash what has been stated time and again previously. People living with Cancer, with MS, AIDS, dementia, with Chronic Pain, need to conserve their energy in as many ways as possible in order to live their best lives in richer and more productive ways by utilizing as many resources that are possible, rather than be exposed to external stressors that only heighten stress and pain.

The mind/body/spirit gives us new and old ways to deal with pain; and it may be that through all our senses we can find creative strategies to enhance coping skills for dealing with pain and its many dimensions.

The kaleidoscopes of colors have never been more stunning as we research and practice the healing powers of the brain/body/spirit connections of healing through imagery, touch, sound, sight, tastes and smells in work of loss, grief, mourning, and pain.

These lenses of color and shape can add to a person's quality of life and ability to withstand pain and suffering at times increasing the ability to do and be with a greater regard for the preciousness of life itself. And it is in these moments that those suffering from chronic pain are able to journal their thoughts and feelings, while recording the very things that work best when they have flare-ups or exacerbations of pain that is best controlled by methods they have learned or taught to others to provide relief.

Below are some "HOW TO" ideas and tips that may help for those living with chronic pain and assist loved ones in helping along the journey:

"How can I get there" asked Dorothy. "You must walk. It is a long journey, through country that is sometimes pleasant and sometimes dark and terrible. However, I will use all the magic arts I know of to keep you from harm."
(The Wizard of Oz)

Yes, sometimes it feels as though you are Dorothy or perhaps one of the many characters she found along the journey, but may you find HOPE in knowing that you are also Oz…. you have all the magic arts within, to facilitate healing from within, to lessen the pain that comes with the fierceness and beauty of lightning and thunder as it courses through your body. You can find ways to protect you, to shield you and to ease some of the pain, with mindfulness, with practice, and with focus.

Through choices that are yours to make and amazing grace, those with chronic pain report that their quality of life improve by using as many alternatives to healing that they can muster and practice in addition to traditional medical interventions. Chronic pain and those who suffer it; each have stories to tell, paths that are uncertain and suffering that is chronic comes at a cost that affects and infects all.
We must learn to see with different eyes, to listen with all our senses as we learn ways to fight the monster that lives under the beds of so many and rears its head so often.

When traditional modalities fail to give those all that is needed; it is time to pull out all the stops and step out of comfort zones and into creativity in order to tap into the Universal energy of ways to help those who suffer as together we fight the monster under the bed.

1. Journaling: journaling dates back to perhaps at least the 10th century! It is a marvelous way to keep track of where you have been, where you are and where you hope to go, and the research has pointed to the increased benefits of journaling in regards to health and growth.

As we've read the journals or diaries of famous and successful people and Presidents, many have also been honored to see or have read the journals of those who kept journals of their most difficult journey through times of great illness, end of life and pain filled times through journals or recordings.

University of Texas at Austin psychologist and researcher, James Pennebacker; contended that journaling decreases the symptoms of asthma and rheumatoid arthritis. He believed that writing about stressful events in one's life helps to come to oneness with the stress, therefore reducing the impact on physical health and well-being.

For those who are grieving, many state that the use of a journal is a great way to record their journey; a tool of healing. For the person in chronic pain, it can be a tool of diversion, yet a tool of empowerment for one to record their thoughts on pain, on loss, on creative ways to incorporate the pain into the life of pain.

Those experiencing pain also experience secondary losses brought about by the limitations placed on them. They can come to terms with the secondary losses by finding adaptive responses to the pain and perhaps find place the pain at bay for a while. This will allow the endorphins to take over while empowering the person in ways not before imagined. By changing the focus of their attention, they can help create a pain free zone, or a pain lowered state.

A journal is also a great barometer as we forget how we have been doing; one can look back two weeks; two months and see how we were, in our own hand, our own mood, our own writing or how far we have come, or yet have to go…. It is also a great place a blank canvas if you will, to dream.

2. Energy work: is a general term for those alternative modalities of working through illness/disease/chronic pain that are based on the idea that the human body consists of energy fields that can be stimulated through varied techniques in order to alleviate pain and promote wellness.

The concept of energy as a healing modality sees energy as a vital life force and can be traced back to the oldest of medical systems. Many cultures use this concept such as Native Americans, the Chinese, the Japanese, the Indians and all around the world in Eastern Medicine and healers.

Healing Energy is based on the concept that every living thing has an energy field that must be balanced in order to maintain proper mental, physical and spiritual health. Illness, including chronic pain occurs when this energy field is either blocked or weakened over time; and one can see the toll on the faces of those who suffer and those who love them. Many will embrace or try acupuncture from licensed practitioners for pain or chronic conditions; and acupuncturists in the USA must be licensed to practice.

3. **Reiki:** is now being used as one of the many and varied alternative treatment modalities of those suffering chronic pain, life threatening illnesses in the world and can be done hands on or from a distance through the use of energy work.

As we know Chronic pain affects millions; their lifestyles, abilities to do and be and enjoy the activities of daily life that so many take for granted. This pain may all of a sudden disappear and then return for no obvious reason, or just find itself at home in one's body and life forever necessitating that person to find and utilize as many ways and means for relief as possible; opening up the mind, body and spirit to take advantage of healing modalities both near and far.

In opening up channels between a patient and one who is adept at Reiki to transfer energy; healers are able to restore balance both physically and mentally. Muscles are able to become relaxed and the energy flow is unblocked for the one suffering chronic pain and illness.

Although the patient may not be pain or disease free, he or she may experience relaxation, a respite from the pain and stress associated with it by that opening up of channels that are blocked from tension and body tightness through that transfer of energy.

Since the early 1990's research has demonstrated that Reiki treatment can and does significantly reduce fatigue, pain and anxiety while improving the overall quality of life for those who suffer pain, suffering and effects secondary to cancer and stress. It is believed to be a result of the "re-balancing" of energy in areas of the body that is experiencing disease and discomfort; while allowing patients to gain better control of their pain and reduce their feeling of being out of control and enhancing their coping mechanisms.

4. **Guided Imagery:** There is tremendous healing energy in imagery for those who suffer chronic pain/suffering along with trauma, life threatening illness and stress. Guided imagery is a relaxation technique(s) that uses narratives to "take you" somewhere in your mind/body/spirit... and ultimately away from the pain that has you in its grip.

I have seen the benefits of these techniques with those who are suffering; those who are dying, those who are grieving as people are able to press on through their lives and increase their abilities to enhance their lives and activities of daily living while increasing their coping mechanisms.

Many will benefit from having someone to lead them in a guided imagery; to listen to a tape as they find their way into the world of relaxation techniques, later to be able to master this and move onto areas of self-imagery for pain control and decreasing stress.

Guided imagery affects the emotional center of the brain; which in turn affects and controls the perceptions of pain for those who are suffering as it speeds healing and affects every aspect of the body.

In guided imagery, you are led by someone's voice, focusing on instructions, on something specific; you are asked to control your breathing while thinking about or concentrating as you are taken on a specific journey if you will, or to a place that allows you to relax. That something, or someplace is often dependent on your goals, on what you need at the time; pain relief, stress relief; perhaps visualizing a stream or mountain top to release the pain or cells of illness or to strengthen your immune system.

These messages and visualizations that are sent to the brain then travel to your immune system, to the autonomic nervous system that affect your heart rate, your blood pressure, your breathing rate, while allowing you relaxation, releasing natural endorphins for pain relief and muscle relaxation along with teaching you enhanced coping skills.

There are proven health benefits of guided imagery that now let us know it is an alternative to traditional interventions and readily available. One can ask for a loved one to record or send videos to those suffering chronic pain for the soothing sounds and guided relaxation.

5. Breathing: Yes we know that breathing is a good thing! It is involuntary for the most part; however most people do not concentrate on their breath. Rather than breathing mindfully, those in pain find that they breathe short gasping breaths between jagged pained periods. It is then that a helpful reminder of slowing ones' breath and taking mindful breaths is helpful.

As a caregiver, one might want to aide in this cautiously and remind the pain sufferer of breathing slowly through the nose, and then exhaling through the mouth as if blowing out candles on a birthday cake... At times it may be difficult; a person in pain does not usually like to be told how to breathe, nor has tolerance for being told "what or how to do", but once reminded to be mindful or to put the oxygen on, they can and will control their breathing which may assist in decreasing their pain and allow them to once again experience enhanced sense of control.

There are many and varied breathing exercises for those in pain; yet when one has pain ranging from 5-8 they will often forget that which they know as pain takes over the brain, body, spirit. Mindful breathing exercises and learning new patterns that become second nature allows us to "imagine" healing is occurring with each breath.

By focusing on breathing, one can allow the body to relax, which will often deter the pain as the body finds its
focus on the breath and endorphins are released by the brain as anxiety is decreased and control sense is increased.

When one is asked/instructed to breathe deeply, it may help to remember, what is "deep breath" to one, is not deep breath to all. Breathe what is comfortable to you without hyperventilating. [Example: "Pay attention to your breathing, without trying to change it: Breathe IN… Breathe out. Notice how quickly or slowly you are breathing. (Pause)… Now notice how shallow or deeply you are breathing as you read this. (Pause)… OK, now pay attention to where your breath is coming in to your body… and where it leaves your body. (pause) Finally, just continue to breath, you now know mindful breathing and what and how you breathe."

Many will meditate, practice yoga if their bodies will allow it. Interestingly, I have found that there are many who reject the word "meditation" and as a result will build up "blocks" and put off what is a simple ritual of healing. It may be that words are so powerful for some we need to re-wire words with negative connotations in order to work through the fear or blocking of action in order to do things that we want.

Words are powerful. For one woman who is a chronic pain sufferer who spent 8 months talking about not being able to focus on meditations; we re-worked her thinking about it; by changing her vocabulary. She now has replaced the word "meditate" with "beauty". Now each day she sits and gazes upon fresh flowers and mindfully breathes, enjoying the view with each breath. She now no longer uses the word "meditate", she is practicing "beauty" daily!

6. Reading: "On a sultry summer night, the wind seemed lifeless and the pain was through the tin roof as I waited for pain and rain to wash me clean;"

Yes, reading can be balm for the soul and can educate on ways to enhance our lives or to deter our minds away from pain, stress and strain. There are a myriad of books, self-help, comedy, drama, and just silliness out there for those of us working with and living with chronic pain, suffering, loss and grief.

Reading is a wonderful way to submerge yourself and move from within and focus shifting from the monster under your bed for a while. Perhaps shifting the focus to those monsters under the beds of others is just what the doctor ordered!

7. Tapes: A great medium available to listen to books, to music, to imagery now available to most people with ear buds so that you can be in control of the volume. Those with chronic pain are often "sound sensitive", often do not want others to necessarily hear or be privy to conversations or tapes that they may be listening to for or about self-help in their beds or homes. We now live in a world where books, imagery work is available by tape, by IPOD, by players and speakers do not have to broadcast the sound loud and for all to hear.

As we mention journaling; it is also a wonderful way to journal by use of a recorder, to record the journey, to leave a legacy for family, for friends when pain is high or low. To keep a journal that later you can play back to see where you are in relation of where you have been and chart the waters of where you hope to go.

The value of taping and listening to tapes is great, healing properties to add to the toolbox of alternatives of healing ways and empower individuals to take charge of their health plan. Also a great idea to take those little $19.95 voice activated recorders to MD appointments in order to record all that is said during those stressful appointments.

It is remarkable how our memory fails us when we are on tables and without clothing as doctors and nurses speak to us; often standing over us, and they are fully clothed. It may be that it is quite empowering to have one of those trusty recorders to listen to once in the safety of our home with our clothes on after those appointments and our senses are regained: the threat and the fears behind us.

8. Music: The healing properties of music go back to the beginning of time. When all else fails; music is the Universal connection to the soul, the spirit, the heart, body and the brain. Music moves people; from their soul; from children to the Elders, folks in wheel chairs and on Canadian crutches will find a way to tap their toes or pat their hands if they like the music! It's been that way since the first drum beat, and research has demonstrated that those with chronic pain report relief; those who are stressed or those who are tense will lighten up with music.

The type of music does not seem to matter as much as the music seems to make people feel better. Those who are in nursing homes, those who are demented are known to sing with music from their era even if they have not spoken two words in years!

Music can and does make a difference in the lives of people at all stages of their lives across the life span. There are times that pain will exist no matter what you throw at it, or what you put in your body; times when you will defy gravity in your ability to move beyond what is reasonable in the eyes of others.

There are times when you may be in your bed with pain that seems off all charts known to man; but a song may come on and you find that your soul will not allow you to be still. OR, you may have to be still, but your spirit will dance as you see yourself dancing across the room in your mind, and all of a sudden your pain begins to lessen and you feel more hopeful than you have inn days as you experience some respite from what has been unrelenting horrific pain.

Music may just speak to the spirit and thereby give a person in pain a sense of greater control and hope through each note, each word that is sung. Music may allow the brain to release endorphins to fight pain and to dance in a bed or against the shadows on the walls and distract a person and attention away from pain for a while.

Slow music and thought provoking music may allow breathing a chance to slow down and restore the body taking over the pain and allow the muscles to relax and refuel by the passion of the music and heal the cells. The wonders of the Universal Connection are not to be ignored.

9. Water: We all know the benefits of water; and when one is in pain or on the go, we seem to never get enough water in us. We need water; we can also be soothed by water, the sounds of water, the healing energy of water.

Those in chronic pain often are also dehydrated! Check with your physician on any water restrictions and if there are none? Drink! Drink! Drink! You need water to run on. Sit a bowl of water by the bedside, dip your fingers in it at times and watch the ripple effect of it; put a beautiful stone in the water, use it well as a reminder to breathe, to be and to take your time.

Knowing that those with chronic pain must take each day, each moment planning how and where to spend their precious energy, it may help to use that stone as a grounding moment. To take it in hand, feel its strength and wet before making the decision of what and how you will move into the day. Place it back in the bowl and see the effects, knowing that your steps will have larger effects on you, those you love and of course there will be a physical price to pay for what you plan and what you do... Be gentle with yourself and ask others to do the same.

10. Ritual: We engage in rituals each and every day. Before our feet hit the floor a ritual is occurring; it may be the way we open our eyes; the thanks we give to our Creator to see another day; the way we stretch into morning; the way we put on slippers, the way we stand and move to the bathroom to brush our teeth! Rituals are time limited structured activities.

Rituals are important and many traditions we hold sacred are rituals today as they have been throughout history. Incorporating rituals into healing ways and life with chronic pain are equally important to enhance coping and quality of life. Many rituals within family systems are now fragmented as families no longer live close together; other rituals within families get strained with life and chronic illness/pain.

 Life becomes more spontaneous rather than planned as those with chronic pain/illness never know how the next day or next week will be; will they be able to attend or cook that favorite meal or participate in ways that once were so paramount. Will they be a disappointment to others, or others want more than they are able to give when pain or the monster comes out from under the bed?

Rituals get disturbed, families and friends get tense, the one in such pain feels diminished and is no longer as it once was. Communications need to med or what be opened and new rituals and traditions started; it becomes a time for Christmas in July at times; spur of the moment celebrations when times are not so awful and one is feeling pretty good!

It's hard to plan when one is chronically ill; and yet life goes on as those dates seem to stay on the calendar and some plans cannot be changed. Life as one with illness or pain or impending death also changes drastically as does the lives of those who love them. Accommodations can be made in all cases with a bit of creativity and an ample dose of understanding! A bed available when the one who is ill grows tired or has a flare; loving friends or family in the next room that understand and continue on knowing that once the crisis passes the person will return to the group.

New rituals in understanding and open communications are all that is needed to decrease stress and allow the chronic pain sufferer to know that they are valued and understood. Rituals and traditions are an important thread in the tapestry of our lives and continue to evolve into newness while holding strong many of the old ways and making necessary changes for those we care for and about.

Families and friends have repetitive interactions and it is those patterns that will regulate behaviors for many. They are the implicit rules for the activities of daily living and often may be "rituals" yet are not often told to each other! But once a member of the family becomes disabled by chronic illness or pain, those rules can change significantly and leave the entire system off balance, requiring all to come together and find new ways and systems to now develop new rituals and new rules to live stronger and together in finding adaptable ways that include all.

It is a time of tremendous challenge and of great growth once communications are open within the family and the person who is suffering enlists supports when addressing the medical communities as well. Change is an ongoing process; and hope is eternal in addressing chronic pain and the monster under the bed beyond traditional medical models.

STORIES OF OTHERS FIGHTING PAIN

Bessie's House:

Having just arrived from 109 degree heat, my shirt was stuck to my back, as I was greeted by a daughter who looked once again like she hadn't slept in days; the house a mess and the offer of coffee was just one more time of offering mindlessly as she already had my cup in her hand.

I smiled and took my coffee, thanking her and taking an inventory around me of the organized chaos of what once was a lovely home before illness had hit wide open and personal. *"She's in her room and hasn't been civil for two days, good luck!"* the daughter said but I could tell she would like to sit a while, so I made a mental note to spend some time with the daughter after my time with Bessie.

As I walked to the bedroom I knew Bessie was aware I was there although she had her back to me; then I heard it; *"Lawd, chile, get in here quick and lock the door!"*. I had to grin, as I walked in the room, but I left the door open a bit, as I am sure her daughter heard her as well.

Bessie was an elderly woman, full of spirit she was, and a woman who in her 90's could still move around with the aid of a cane unless she was upset with someone (which she was a lot these months), then she would forget the cane. She was a real spit fire Bessie was and today would prove to be no exception to that rather remarkable assessment. Bessie was dressed today; had her back to me and was facing the bed when I arrived. She was known to have severe pain issues and at times was confined to her bed; while at others would be in such pain that one only had to look at her face and wonder how she could dress and walk at all.

She was always kind to me; at times asking that I just sit with her or listen to music as she told me stories and shared her life in an intimate way as if we were old friends from a time long ago. She and her daughter were close, but oh they had moments of high heat as Bessie would let go and release her pent up anger on that child of hers.

Patients and those in pain often will strike out on those that are closest to them, at times over the most ridiculous of things. Sandwiches that are not cut kiddy-corner but straight across comes to mind on this day as a horrible act committed by a faithful and kind caregiver who was exhausted.

As I approached the bed to give Bessie her ritual hug of hello, she turned on a dime like she was expecting change! In her hand was a knife as she wielded it and hollered, *"did you lock that door for me and where have you been?"* I was not prepared for my old friend Bessie this morning as I almost dropped my coffee in surprise of this greeting of hers, and saw in her eyes that she was in tremendous pain. I simply said, *"Well, good morning to you my sweet Ms. Bessie, this is not your usual greeting! What in the world are you doing pointing your knife at me today?"* With that I could hear footsteps and the daughter arrived with a shriek, *"Mama what in the hell you doing with that knife?"*

Well that was probably not the best next thing, given I could see the pain in Bessie's eyes and the knife was pointed at me, my coffee was about to spill and I was hot.

So as Bessie began to let loose her hollering and all hell about to bust loose, I really just wanted to sit down and enjoy my coffee with my old friend; after all it was in my plan for the day. Poor Bessie had been up all night, her pain off the chart and almost beyond her own ability to cope. *"Get her out of this room, didn't I tell you to lock the door, I've been waitin for you to get here, now scoot, make her leave NOW".*

Well, when Ms. Bessie speaks one needs to pay attention, so I sat down my coffee, cautiously backed up to the daughter and told her everything was going to be just fine. I asked her to just go and have some coffee and toast; we would be alright here. She was worried, it was evident. I had asked her if Ms. Bessie had her medications for pain, and she said *"Let me go and get them. I'll be right back".*

I then told Ms. Bessie that I would lock that door after I got the medications for her pain and saw with my own eyes her take them and asked if we had a deal. She grinned that little wicked grin of hers and said, *"Well alright but I want some coffee too then"*. OK, we can do that and I let the daughter know with repeating that out the door with one eye on Bessie as I waited.

Once the daughter returned I brought the pills and coffee to Bessie who then had me to put them in her mouth and took the coffee to down them. She was a sly one alright as it then allowed her to keep that blade in the other hand. She kept her part of the bargain, so I again backed to the door and told the daughter to go and rest as we are good here, and locked me in with Bessie,

As I returned to the bed where she was standing with that gleaming old knife I then asked her again, "so why the knife greeting my friend?" I leaned over the knife and gave her a kiss on the cheek. She smiled her sweet smile and said these words that I will forever keep with me; a lesson to be shared.

"I've been in such pain that I would have to die to feel better. I knew my daughter would just say I'm a crazy ole woman, but you, well you are different. So I've been waiting all night for you to get here, and I got up and made myself get dressed, found my old knife here. I just knew if you got here you would help me. My mother once told me if you take your sharpest knife and put it between the mattress it will cut the pain, so I been waiting for you chile to help me lift this mattress up so I can place it. You see it won't help if you place it because it ain't your pain. I been having my back to the door so she won't see me with it cos she so nervous bout me I just know she would end up calling the police or something saying I'm crazy... I've had to be holding this knife to put me into it, so when I place it, this knife will cut it. You with me on this now?"

I listened with all my senses, her eyes never moved from mine, her hands steady as a rock as she held that knife with its silver shining and its point at times near me; her words made such sense in a world that little makes sense and many are never listened to.

"Yes Ms. Bessie, I am with you my friend, I understand and I am so sorry I was late getting to you. Are you ready to do this right now?" I helped her up, and she stood by as I lifted that mattress up and she placed that knife exactly where she wanted it to be, and then sat it back carefully as she instructed me. I then helped her sit back down comfortably and we had our coffee for a long time in silence before she then shared with me the story handed down by her mother and her mother's mother on that knife that cut the pain.

I watched as her eyes and skin transformed into a woman who felt more in control, her laughs became easier, her eyes filled with tears at one point and said she was so old, that when she died she would have to hire pallbearers as everyone she once knew had already died. We talked and I sat beside her on the bed, with one hand on hers; it was soft; it had seen and felt much in 90 years of life.

We talked about the importance of staying ahead of the pain with her medications; of remembering that her daughter is doing the best she can; and cannot always remember the angle of cutting that egg salad sandwich but is trying her best. Bessie said, *"At times I look at her and think of all the times of hers I am taking and feel so bad for her, it wasn't spose to be this way... I'm takin too much of her time you know"*.

She felt sad and bad about that; as I then wondered if we could invite the daughter into our locked room, I rather imagined she was leaning against the door wondering if I had been bludgeoned by Bessie. I swear that woman was reading my mind as she said, "Wonder if she thinks I stabbed you yet? Guess we should invite her in before she kills herself looking through the keyhole. Walk softly and open it and let's see if she falls in will you chile."

I thought I would laugh myself silly with the thought, but I did as she asked and sure enough there was a loving daughter who almost fell through the opened door as I pulled it. We all got a great laugh from that, and she joined us with fresh coffee and a story that had her crying on how one with chronic pain wanted to cut pain but was afraid she would not be understood.

JEREMY SAYS:

Chronic pain is not for the faint of heart, not for those who cannot stand for their feelings to be hurt from time to time, or for their boxes not to be stretched every now and again.

Jeremy was 13 and had big dreams; to ride a Harley, to work in a sky rise building, to Jet Ski, to be 16 and go to the prom.... And then came the pain; the chronic pain that stopped all that, and the changes in the family, the fights, the drama, the tears and the fatigue; and the pain medications that did not help the pain as much as it altered his moods and made him sleepy and grumpy.

"Why are you here and what do you want from me?" The words of a kid who just did not want another stranger in his home asking dumb questions nor offering suggestions, taking an assessment, or trying to make sense of things that just do not make sense.

At times it really sucks to be in the helping professions when you just are at a loss for words for those who are in pain; those whose futures do not hold bright and sterling dreams nor lives that seem to have meaning for them or those that love them.

As I pulled up a chair and introduced myself, I knew it would be a short visit, as I was about to be thrown out of this young ones room, I could feel it coming. Meet Jeremy, a 13 year old who was racked in pain and on enough pain medicine to stop a moose at 50 yards, yet with a quick wit and not a lot of room for B.S., and he had already met a host of those professionals in the helping field that he had made sure Mom had fired or he had himself. Would I be next?

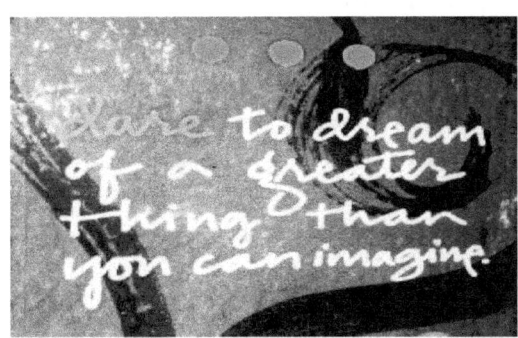

I remembered a kid once told me the best way to open the door is to not talk about stuff that is not easy to understand; skip all that I was told, and "just talk like I matter to you, like a real person". No one wants to hear "psycho-babble" or techie terms of illness and such; they want to hear from your heart to their heart, so I just needed to "think 13".

That was a lifetime ago; so let me start with the sky rises, that would be easy. As I glanced at this kid my heart ached; he was thin, pale, and in remarkable pain as his brow was furrowed, his fists clenched and jaw set as if fighting someone in armor with a sword. I bucked up and said, "So why the fascination with sky rises?" He stared at me for the longest time and then laughed out loud.

He finally said, "I like you Showalter; that is the funniest thing anyone has ever said to me so far. Actually NO ONE has ever asked me about anything but how are you feeling; what do you think about when you feel like this, do you know you will never ride a Harley or a bicycle again? Those are the usual questions until now!" Ok, we have a start point and I like that he called me "Showalter". Ok I think I will like this pain filled kid as well.

The mother had heard him laugh and came into the room with a puzzled look on her face, glanced at him, then at me. She asked if all was ok, and then grinned and left quickly. Jeremy then went on to tell me about his fascination about sky rises and while he was talking I witnessed his brow ease some, his fists start to relax a bit, although I knew he was in considerable pain.

At one point he stopped to ask if I would mind re-filling his water and also bringing him his meds from his Mother if I had the time to stay. I assured him we were "all good" and left the room to let Mom know I thought I had passed the test, and got what he asked for, along with a cup of coffee. She was surprised but no more than I was, as I returned to this old soul. We then began a friendship and he took me on a journey of pain through the eyes of a 13 year old and ways to move through pain by imagination and strategy.

Jeremy and I would have many visits together, usually twice a week where I introduced him to guided imagery and he was eager and ready when I arrived. We would begin with an update and him showing me his latest and greatest posters and pictures of sky rises, Harleys and share dreams he had.

From there we would prepare him for guided imagery after doing touch to relax him. He had a gentle touch, and would ask if he could check my pulse to match it with his; to determine his rate against mine and later to determine if guided imagery had changed either his or mine.

He was open to the benefits of touch and imagery and used a pain scale, a journal of imagery that he would look at as night fell, in order to relax him with music. His mom reported a change in him; decreased pain over all, increased satisfaction in his interactions within the family and with his little sister. They shared more time when he was in his bed; talking, spending time as a family.

Harsh words seemed to not be as frequent as he had found an outlet to his frustrations; and he now asked for massage from his mom; talked to her about imagery and checked her pulse against his to determine if she and he were calm before and after doing imagery and talk together.

He found ways to compliment the traditional paths of medicine he was receiving and he self-reported needing less medicine than before utilizing talk therapy and visualizations. Jeremy began allowing friends to visit again; was introduced to a group from Rolling Thunder the motorcycle group that rides for Memorial day into Washington D.C. and was able to ride with them and he was thrilled.

On a day when his pain was not too intense, he was taken to the top of a sky rise building and had lunch, but once he saw so many in those suits and fast pace from on top of a roof top he thought maybe that was not for him, as he had felt the wind on his face and the sun and roar of thunder.

He was a gift that continued to provide lessons for all in the profession to learn from when approaching his bedside and remembering to learn all that is possible before the introductions and jumping into disease and illness with real talk before the scary stuff in an effort to provide holistic care.

Jazz and the Pain:

Jazz will not often tell you how bad she is hurting. You must look into her eyes to see. On those very rare occasions where she does tell you, it is comments like these:

"Oh please help me this pain is killing me... I feel like I am being tortured."

"I feel like lightning bolts going through my body and searing me"

"Fire is soaring through my veins and God I am miserable".

And when you look at her face and into her eyes, you can tell she is traveling through that hell called severe chronic pain. My sweet friend Jazz has been a chronic pain sufferer for years; her pain being treated poorly by a health care professional that did not seem to get it. Her health history could stretch from one end of a hallway to the other; yet each visit she would be made to sit in uncomfortable chairs and wait.

Jazz is stoic and her usual response is "I am fine" and she will smile or joke. She says that is her choice and while she is still able to choose that is what she wants to do. I have learned that the more she jokes, the worse her pain really is.

Her pain can be so horrible that just to make the doctor appointment would boggle the mind; yet the scheduling desk was sure to remind to be there on time; however once there, no considerations were made to make this person comfortable or the provider to be prompt.

It seems the medical times have changed and seeing the doctor is not something patients like Jazz get to do often for many doctors no long like to do Medicaid or Medicare and so, she must suffer with Physician's Assistants and sometimes not very good ones or very caring ones. Pain takes the strength of a warrior.

Yes, it is times like this that one would like to scream and bang their head against the wall as they write to their congressman and

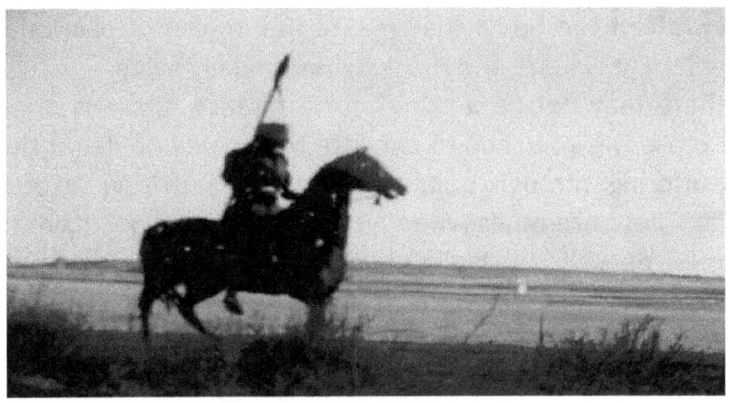

the American Medical Association demanding that someone STAND UP for patients and advocate for justice. Chronic pain untreated or treated improperly invades the body, spirit, soul and erodes a person's resiliency.

Jazz was in pain that no one should have to experience in this time and age of medical break trough's as we can put folks into space, make cars run without gasoline and do all sorts of remarkable things within the body and detect cells neurotransmitters in the brilliance of the brain.

Yet, a Physician's Assistant who should be really concentrating on those with colds and flu is allowed to practice medicines on a person with complex medical conditions; and at that provide poor and substandard care. Why is this?

People must find ways to empower themselves and to demand to be cared for and seen by those who are knowledgeable in the field of medicine, while finding the energy or asking their caregivers to draft letters to those in power to know about when things are just wrong. There are times when Jazz is rendered unable to move from her hospital bed secondary to pain that is excruciating. Thankfully this is a woman who is open to receive the many alternatives to compliment traditional and even poor care while attempting to survive and find better care.

Many chronic pain sufferers would be wise to investigate, to get an informational visit from a Palliative Care Specialist around the country. They are the "true pain experts" and know exactly how medications affect the body; they realize the impact of pain on the person, the family system, and the activities of daily living.

While there may not be a "cure" for a disease, there is often a way to decrease the pain, and to enhance the quality of life for those who are suffering through pain management, nutrition, exercise, adaptations. There are times when Jazz is in so very much pain; that she has to "dig deep" in the well to find the will to fight.

It is during those times that touch is important; gentle massage, a hand to hold, and reassuring words of comfort. Words are powerful tools, and those words must be mindful. One will never ever know exactly what one with chronic pain is living through; not even another person with chronic pain.

Jazz would often message me and say "Please, I need energy work" and we would do it by phone or Skype. Jazz was sensory enough that she could close her eyes and feel my hands running down her legs to pull the painful energy out even with distance between us.

I remember one night that I was doing energy work on her legs. Jazz was not a patient but a friend who suffered severely with pain who turned to me to help her. I could hear her talking as I was going through the energy motions and I was talking to her as I did it. Suddenly she told me that she could visualize the Indian Chief beside me doing the same motions. Jazz also had Native American in her and for her to say this did not shock me. I kept working and talking until finally I heard her say "I can breathe now. It is ok"

Jazz later told me that when she was doing visualization when the pain was high and she could not get hold of me, that she saw the Indian Chief working over her legs that would spasm like a contortionist. She said the Chief would look into her eyes and motion shhhh and continue working on her legs. The mind is powerful if we allow it to be and Jazz was exceptional in that she allowed all of her senses to work and could smell the sage I burned from home from her hospital bed. And when she said she visualized the Indian Chief, she said she could smell the sage and herbs burning in the room.

Pain is whatever a person says it is; and each is individual and different. Perception is reality for many and stronger than reality for

34

many more. At times, one who is in a flare or pain crisis only need to know there is someone who cares. Not someone who says, "I know just how you feel", nor "I can fix this", "what do you want me to do", "let me know if I can do anything" or other similar phrases.

Those with chronic pain do not know what they want or need another to do, but they do know that no one knows how they feel, nor can anyone fix it. At times and as hard as it is to realize, many things are beyond the control of others; and another's pain is one of them. Pain is like the grief of another or our own pain for that matter at many times.

That is another piece of the pain; it makes us feel out of our own control, which is painful on many levels. It is a form of grief to be one who suffers daily with chronic health issues and pain. Those who do are suffering by inches and grieving losses daily from what was, should be, could have been and how it might have been if only...

Jazz will employ creative techniques after being one who knows the path of a chronic pain sufferer over many years. She will turn down the volume, turn down the lights, turn up self-soothing modalities and hold tight to faith. Those who have a strong faith foundation handle pain, loss, grief, and healing much better than those who are without.

She has been another with great lessons and lives with jazz, spark, even at times when the lights are low, her internal light is bright as she continues to fight for the care she deserves and the monster under the bed to leave town if only for a while. How she has remained so sweet and kind with so much pain I will never know. I just know she has remained a dear and loyal friend to me and shows care for everyone in spite of her horrific pain.

ThunderBolt in The HOUSE:

It was about 10:00 pm when the phone rang, and I dreaded that call. I had a sense it was my beautiful elderly friend who had been on hospice care for more than a year. She was in her 80's had been so frail, in such awful pain and weak over the last couple of months.

I had laughed a few months earlier while visiting her when she told me if she could have it all she would have fresh clean sheets on her bed every day and fresh flowers in her house to look at each day of her life. She was bright as the sun, and we had such grand times. I remembered saying to her, "Well I cannot do those sheets every day, but I can promise you the fresh flowers will be here dear lady"!

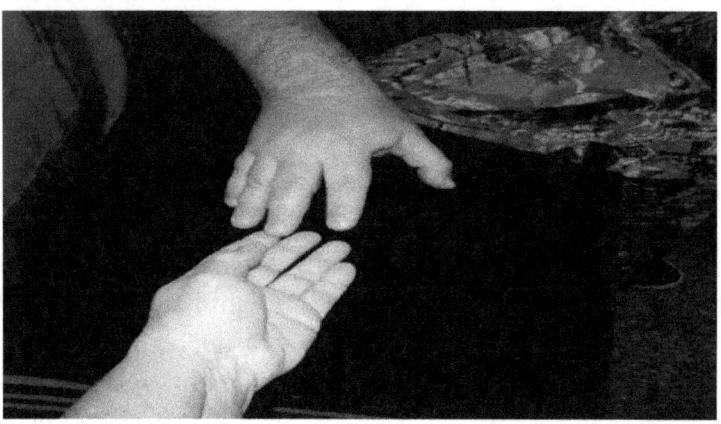

So it was with a certain dread I picked up the phone, only to hear the weak voice of my sweet Thunderbolt on the other end of the phone, "Did I wake you? I think I need you". Oh that voice sounded weak, no thunder did I hear in that call, as I assured her I would be right there as soon as I got out of the jammies and brushed my hair.

On my way there I kept thinking about the last few months; and wondered did she say she needed me or it was getting close... I could not remember, but I did know how weak she sounded. Maybe I should stop by McDonalds for her a chocolate milkshake as she sure loves those. What am I thinking?? My friend could have been calling to say I am dying and in pain, get your ass over here, and I am thinking about milkshakes???

Wonder if I should call her "Thunderbolt" like I always have when I get there tonight; oh brother, where did she hide the key to get in the house? Questions; I seemed to be filled with questions as I drove through the dark to get to the house. Seems we are never ready to say so long to a friend and yet, I knew she had fought so long with such pain.

As I pulled into the driveway I knew one thing to be sure, I was glad she had the strength to call me; was ever so glad there was and had been fresh flowers there ever since she made that desire known. And now it was time for me to find that key wherever it was and get inside. Sure hope she does not ask me why I did not stop for the milkshake tonight.

As I bent down to look under the mat, the door swung opened and I caught a familiar smell of Chanel #5 and almost fainted. There she stood in her little outline in her robe; and motioned me in. Oh, she was so weak and frail, and I could tell by her shaky hug she was in pain.

"Get in here before someone grabs you in the dark". I found myself laughing out loud as I said, "Thunderbolt you scared me half to death. What are you doing answering the door". She took my hand and led me to the couch unsteady on her feet as she said, "Well I figured you wouldn't remember the key, and where is my milkshake honey?" I just knew it!

So I hugged her but did not want to hurt her and said, "Well I thought you were dying and did not want to take time to get it. What is wrong that you have me out here tonight?" She then looked at me through those crystal blue piercing eyes and said, "Oh, I've been in so much pain honey, and I'm on that pain patch. I've taken enough morphine to kill a horse and I think it's time. Have you got any money?"

Ok, I am playing this in my mind; she is on a pain patch, has taken enough morphine to render a horse dead, which means she should be unconscious or sound asleep or slurring her words or something. And she has just busted me for not bringing the milkshake. Now she thinks it is time. But, why is she asking me if I have any money? As I watched my dear friend I realized my mind was going a million miles a minute as the neurotransmitters were trying to process all the information I was hearing, the sights I was looking at and smelling her fragrance toppled with the beauty of the flowers in her wonderful home.

She just gazed at me with a wicked sort of grin and asked me again, "well do you have any money?" as she patted my hand tenderly and then reached up to stroke my bewildered looking face meeting me eye to eye. I stuttered at that point if I recall and felt my pocket and said, "Well Thunderbolt, I think I have a little money; do you need some? And what do you mean it is time?" I was holding her hands in mine as she told me to help her up. I stood and helped her to rise and she led me through the living room and into the dining room and flipped the light switch.

I stood with my sweet Thunderbolt and looked and there at the table she had transformed it; the table was set for cards, the chips were set, and an ashtray was placed along with three glasses of iced tea. In a couple of minutes here came her husband down the steps and he grinned and said, "Guess she told you didn't she, it's time? Do you have any money?"

I could not believe my eyes or ears. I started to laugh a bit, and could not help myself when I asked, "Are you raising money for the mortgage or the funeral?" They both just laughed themselves silly as they took my money and traded it for chips, as I helped Thunderbolt to her chair still trying to comprehend what was really going on at this table with such a lovely couple.

I did realize that a woman on this cocktail of pain medicine most probably would not be sharp as the usual tack. I noticed that her husband seemed a bit uneasy, yet his jovial self with such love in his gaze of his beloved wife of 58 years as she took the cards in her frail hands and gave me a wink as our late night of cards began.

We talked, we laughed and we took moments between Thunderbolt robbing me blind to talk about going to heaven and seeing so many old friends. We talked about how her beloved husband would fare without her here to nag him, to cuddle with him, and to tell him what colors go best together.

We did a life review as she was still sharp as a tack and let me know that taking all my money had eased her pain better than morphine and she hoped to live long enough to teach me how to play cards a bit better for the next person who might want to keep me up all night for a game of cards.

Yes, my Thunderbolt and her ways to say so long to a friend were quite something as we sat up all night with brief respites for something to eat; me borrowing enough money from her to make a run to McDonalds in the middle of the night for milkshakes and burgers to go with the card game and her to take a wee nap in order to have the strength to continue on.

She suggested I might want to stop by the local ATM machine for a little cash while I was out or she could front me some money but only if I showed up the next day to pay, as time was short and her husband might need the cash and after all she had heard, "I can't take it with me can I?"

Humor in healing ways is and always will be one of the best alternatives to pain pathways and dear sweet Thunderbolt is now riding the lightning I feel certain as she has probably rounded up some card players in the next place where she has no pain.

Tay-Hey:

"Oh please make the pain stop, I can't talk about how I am with pain like this, my head and arms are killing me!!!" As I sat by the bed with this person and the family I felt my stomach in knots, my heart in my mouth and sorrow as deep as the ocean. I watched the family try to sing together, pray together, to make jokes and their voices rise to override the sound of agony from a young man in his 40's in horrible pain.

He screamed; he threw his head from side to side, he cursed like a marine, sailor and all the armed forces out in war at once together in battle as his pain brought tears and jerks to his body and nothing or no one seemed to help him.

We looked to each other as if something magic would come to us at once that we could do to help as we waited for medicine to work its wonder and together we were powerless to do anything but be strong with him. At one point it struck me how tight his muscles were as I saw them strain from pain and the veins pop almost from his skin, revolting from the pain that was searing him.

Tay-Hey screamed for his brother to take his Mom from the room having seen with his eyes the horror his pain was causing her; knowing that he could not prevent the words from escaping from his mouth, but the little bit of control could still protect his lovely mother. And his brother quickly obeyed and you could see his relief in leaving the room with his arm around her as if protecting her from such harsh reality of pain in its glory.

Now there were three of us there including Tay-Hey; and our hearts were breaking as he screamed out his plea of "help me or shoot me now". Tay-Hey a gorgeous man; one arm amputated and phantom pain now searing him; its intensity remarkable, the other arm twitching in recoil to pain while his head throbbing as I watched the veins and could not imagine what he was experiencing.

Suddenly he reached out and grabbed my arm with a grasp that took my breath away. I placed my hand on his and said, "I am here Tay, and I will stay here, just please look at me and breathe with me NOW". Through his tears and ours, we all tried and tried to get him to focus and to concentrate on his breathing. His brother put on drumming music; as we worked and worked on him to focus on his breath.

His father took and folded a long towel and made it attach to where his arm was bandaged after the amputation and rolled it there. Placing it carefully under the covers to look like it extended as the other would; and kept his hand right on that bandage; and kept saying, "son breathe and listen".

For hours we stayed, we chanted, we prayed, we breathed with him. We put ice behind his neck, and we softly talked and had him look directly at us; each of us as we matched his breath with ours. The drums were playing in the background softly as we reminded him that he is a warrior; that he will beat as the drums beat and drum this pain out of him.

His mother and brother returned with steaming cups of hot water they had brought back; and in those cups that had put sage; and its smell was in the room. Tay-Hey could smell it, and he grew quieter, he grip lessoned on my arm, but he kept it there as he breathing slowed and his pain lessoned, we stayed.

As his beloved mother dried his face with a warm cloth dipped in that sage water, he grew more at peace. He knew he was not alone; he knew and believed he would heal and we stayed. Tay-Hey received his prosthesis, was in the care of a pain specialist, and was treated for post-traumatic stress syndrome. He is healing; the drums are beating differently, and he is never alone. People with chronic pain need to know they are not alone.

I have been taught by the real experts on ways to soothe, to ride the rails of pain management, and to each of them I am grateful. Chronic pain is a journey that no one should have to go through alone.

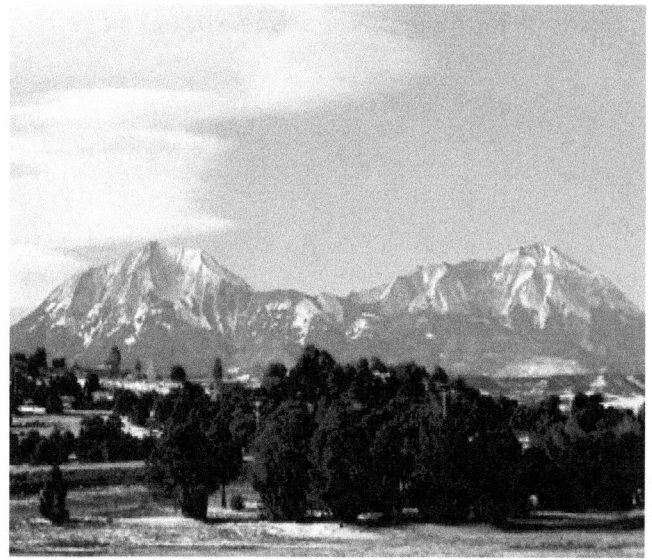

PART TWO

THE MONSTER BENEATH OUR BEDS

Dealing with Chronic Pain from a Caretaker Perspective

By

John Argent

About Chronic Pain

The monster under our beds is that evil entity that sneaks out and wrecks havoc with the lives of those that suffer with chronic pain. That monster is chronic pain. Many people suffer with chronic pain and unfortunately it is handled poorly. Doctors fear addiction and are afraid to prescribe and people suffer. Those who have never suffered chronic pain think they understand but they do not.

It is hard to understand something that takes over your life, keeps you from sleeping, wakes you when you do go to sleep and limits everything you try to do. It is like a monster that comes in and takes away your life. It invades every crevice of your being.

Many will tell those with chronic pain that they know exactly what they are going through but they really have no idea. I have heard people listen to someone who just fell and tore the rotator cuff of their shoulder, had massive inflammation in the shoulder and chest area and were in agony and the person would tell this person in pain that they knew exactly what they felt like as their shoulder hurt like that too, as they were walking out the door to go play tennis.

Please make sure to talk to your doctor before trying any of these. I am not a doctor but rather a caretaker that has worked with chronic pain clients and I also suffer with chronic pain myself. This book is about alternative methods to help a person cope when the pain medicine is not giving the amount of relief we want or need. It is the methods that require us to use our imagination and a willingness to try alternative things. It is not meant to replace what your doctor does but rather to add to it or enhance what the doctor does. Our hope is that these suggestions will give you some relief and help you build emotional tools in dealing with chronic pain for with chronic pain can come depression. The depression makes our pain worse.

We have natural pain killers in our systems called endorphins that can help us ease our pain if we allow our mind and body to use them. Using alternative modalities can often help in this situation. A person with a positive attitude will have greater success with these many alternative methods because they will believe that it works and what the mind believes becomes a reality.

In war situations years ago when they ran out of morphine, they told people that a plain pill like an aspirin was really a new pain medicine that was supposed to be better than morphine. The injured soldiers believed it and because of their belief that this was a great pain medicine, their own endorphins kicked in to help control their pain. The mind can be a powerful thing if we are willing to open it to possibilities and are willing to try alternative things to help with chronic pain.

We have to remember first that pain is necessary. Pain tells us when we are hurting ourselves such as getting too close to the burner on the stove or pushing our muscles beyond what they should be doing. Physical pain, like emotional pain tells us that we need to step back and take another look at what we are doing. It is not the enemy but when it is out of control and chronic, it can be debilitating.

It is important to realize that we will still deal with some pain and that is ok. It is the pain that limits us that we want to find ways to decrease. Because chronic pain is something that invades every part of our lives and affects everything we do, finding ways that work with what our doctor does can help enhance the pain relief we get. When we can help drop the pain or take the edge off of the pain just a little, then we can endure it a little easier.

If you are looking for an instant cure for pain, this is not the book for you. Pain is an integral part of life and we will not be pain free but we can find a more tolerable level of pain if we are willing to allow our minds to help us.

Many people think that a pain pill or anything that is supposed to help pain should remove it totally and become angry and upset when it does not, which only increases their pain. Please keep in mind that we can and should be able to endure a certain amount of pain daily and still enjoy our lives. It is the pain that stops us from carrying on with life that we want to try to tone down.

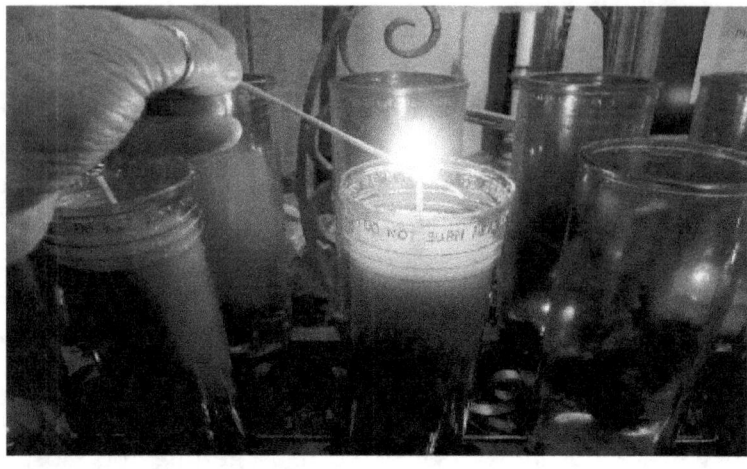

Talking To Your Doctor

Learning to talk to doctors about our pain is extremely important and how we talk to them is crucial. Many people will just tell the doctor that their pain is horrible and when asked to give a number between 1 and 10, some people will say a number like 20 or even 80.

Understanding pain charts can be complicated because none of them actually tell you how to decipher the correct number and if we do not know how to express our pain in a number, then our doctor does not really know how our pain is affecting our lives.

It helps if we can tell the doctor exactly how pain is impacting our lives. For example, is the pain keeping you from doing your normal daily activities? Is it keeping you from enjoying life? Is it keeping you from sleeping or eating? Can you still get up and walk around? Can you walk far? Is it constant? Does it come and go? Where is it? Are you feeling isolated from your pain? Can you dress yourself? Can you go to the bathroom alone?

It is very important to describe your pain by how it impacts your life. Pain can be mild, moderate and severe and each level has to do with how the pain is affecting what you do. Pain becomes debilitating when it affects you daily from normal life activities such as taking care of yourself, dressing, feeding, etc.

What I have learned about pain is that the numbers 1-3 are pain levels that do not affect you much at all. It is pain that after a bit seems to go away because you have become used to it. An example I would use could be like bumping your head. It hurts at first but then the pain seems to subside; it is tolerable pain.

As a caretaker, I found that many people tend to say a higher number than their pain really is because they do not understand how to rate themselves and saying a 5 for example sounds low for how their pain feels when in reality a pain level of 5 is a strong pain that lingers and can interfere to some degree with what you do daily. A pain level of six is a stronger pain that makes you focus most of your energy on getting relief, whether it is taking meds or bed rest or whatever. Knowing how to rate yourself will make it easier for doctors to treat you and hopefully will make your pain management much better.

I hear people say all the time that their pain level is a nine and yet they are up walking around, talking clearly and fixing their own food, taking care of the house or going to the store. A pain level of nine should be so severe that you cannot stand it without narcotic pain killers and many people would even demand invasive procedures to make it stop. A torn rotator cuff in your shoulder comes to mind.

People who rate their pain as a 10 or a 20 or even an 80 when they are capable of walking into the doctor's office and sitting there carrying on a conversation only tend to make doctors think that the pain is not that bad. When you can give a number between one and ten that actually shows what your pain is, then the doctors can see what your pain is really doing to your life. Unfortunately, we have to play by their rules on describing pain or they do not understand.

I live with chronic pain and there are times my pain has put me to bed where I could not get up for a few days and at that time I would say my pain was a 7 because it had effectively disabled me for those few days.

I have learned and try to teach my clients how to not fight pain but rather to use alternative methods to help control their pain. It takes a calm attitude with pain which is hard when you are hurting badly but you can do it. We have to find ways to self soothe ourselves so that we do not overload our senses and thus make the pain worse.

Starting off, the first thing we must do is know what chronic pain is and what it is doing to us and we must learn how to address this with our doctors. If the doctor does not understand what your pain is doing to you, then he cannot effectively treat the pain or offer any alternative methods to use to help with the pain.

One of the most important things to remember is to write down your pain day by day and carry that with you to the doctor. Tell exactly what you were doing for that will help them understand your pain better. For example, does exertion make it worse? Were you lying down or sitting in the recliner and your pain increased? Arthritis is one ailment that inactivity can increase pain, so this is important for your doctor to know. Pain does not come in uniform packages. There are different kinds of pain and different levels of pain.

And the last piece of advice I can give you is that if you get a doctor that is not sensitive to what you have to say, that does not listen, that treats you like you are there just for drugs when you are there for chronic pain, then find another doctor. We deserve to be treated with respect.

Identifying Your Pain Triggers

People have different levels of tolerance to pain and these alternative things can help no matter what level of tolerance you have. As a caretaker, one thing I have noticed about people with chronic pain is that sometimes they fight the pain, which only makes it worse. They become frantic wanting instant relief and then become angry because they do not get it. These negative emotions only stress the system more and make the pain level increase.

A good friend of mine, who lives with chronic pain, told us one day that we should treat chronic pain like it is a good friend. By that, he means we should be gentle with ourselves, not fight it; do special things for it and use every method we can to help soothe the chronic pain. That is a new concept when what we want most is to terminate or destroy this thing called pain but by treating it like a good friend, we lower our stress level which in turn helps to lower our pain level. And we also treat ourselves with greater care and gentleness.

When we are less stressed, when we recognize our limitations and the things that trigger our pain, we are able to cope with our pain a lot better. A trigger is something that increases your pain. Things like stress, financial worries, hectic schedules, relationship problems, and difficulties with children or family members are all things that stress all of us and especially trigger the pain of a person with chronic pain. This book is focusing on things that you can change in your environment, on ways you can treat your pain and yourself and using your mind to help control your pain. While the things mentioned above will increase our pain, they are things that you have to learn how to handle and deal with.

One of the things that I do with my client is listing all of the things in his environment that triggered his pain and made it go higher. His list consists of bright lights, loud noises, heat, crowds, and motion. When we help to control just these few things, it helps his overall pain level. Learning how to recognize your triggers and when you are doing the things that make your pain worse are important parts of learning to be in control of your pain.

The crowd one is obvious. Do not go into big crowded stores, do not have big crowds at home and you can do this by visiting in smaller groups of one or two people rather than a whole family group there and shopping at times when the crowd level is lower.

We decided that the first thing my client should do when his pain rises so high is to go into his bedroom, with the lights very low, with no television or radio playing and a fan on to make the room feel cooler. He lays there on his bed with a cool cloth on his eyes and tries to relax and allow his senses to calm so that he can better deal with the pain.

Loud noises bother my client and so we devised a solution to make the sound of the television and/or computer on a much lower level. Our solution was putting computer speakers on the televisions so that the speaker is right beside his recliner or right beside his hospital bed. He also uses ear buds when the pain is peaking. This makes the room seem more serene and he can put the volume on very low without feeling the painful vibrations of sound that seem to trigger the pain.

Although there is no scientific testing done on this, I believe that people with chronic pain are so sensitive that the vibrations of sound are actually felt in their systems and that is what makes loud noises make their pain higher.

To help with the bright lights triggering pain, we use indirect lighting and have a small lamp by his bed and by his recliner with a higher watt bulb if he needs brighter light to read or work on something. The indirect lighting puts a glow around the room but does not seem harsh and helps soothe his pain rather than antagonize it.

For the heat issue, we use fans around him. The sound of the fan is soothing to him and the gentle breeze blowing over him helps keep his body temperature lower and helps his pain. He has also learned that when his pain is really high, that movement causes his pain to rise so he puts himself on bed rest. While he does not want to lose his muscle by staying in bed all the time, sometimes this is necessary to help him tolerate the higher pain level.

It is very important to remember that your home is for you. Yes, visitors may come but the things you do to help your pain you should do for yourself. If visitors find it different or do not like it, that is their problems. People with chronic pain must take care of their pain first and do the things necessary to reduce pain. It is not being selfish; it is taking care of yourself and your needs. It is hard enough when pain takes away part of our lives but even harder if we try to please everyone and overlook our own personal needs.

Massage and Immobilizing the Painful Areas

Everyone will tell you how good a back massage feels when they are tired and their back is hurting. We do not have to go to a massage therapist to get massage. Sometimes a friend or loved one will do it for us and sometimes we can do it for ourselves. It all depends on where the painful area is.

I recognize that sometimes a person in high pain does not want to be touched because the skin has become so sensitive. Often this is due to dry skin that makes the nerve endings even more sensitive than normal. And so, these steps are based on what you can and cannot tolerate. One of the things my client has learned how to do is self massage, but whether it is massaging your own legs, arms, feet or you have someone to do it for you, it is still one way to help with pain.

A massage does not have to be firm rubbing of the limbs. Touch is an essential part of all of us and sometimes just gently rubbing the hands or arms or shoulders can release tension which will help lower the pain level. Think about how soothing it is when someone rubs our shoulders when we are tired. That soothing feeling for a chronic pain sufferer is something we all want and search for. Massage, even done by yourself, can soothe tired and tense muscles and help them to relax so that you can rest.

Massaging too roughly can cause the muscles to contract and that can increase our pain instead of lowering it, so remember to do it gently and to massage small areas at a time. I have found that rubbing my feet together and over each other often relieves the pain of standing on them and is a self soothing action. There are many massage items out there on the market but you can also use other things that you have right in the house. For example, a can of soup or vegetables placed on the floor and rolling the can back and forth under the arch of your foot it will help ease the spasms of the arch of the foot.

Sometimes we take my clients legs, which give him extreme pain, and after massaging them with herbal oils, we wrap them with ace bandages to hold them from movement and keep the herbal oil close to the skin. After about thirty minutes we remove the bandages. He has actually gotten enough relief that he could doze off after the legs were wrapped.

We have also found that gentle stretching while massaging also helps ease some of the pain. What happens is the more we hurt, the tighter our muscles get and that increases the pain level. Stretching them out gently helps to relax the muscles. Because of muscle loss, the muscles can become spastic and spasm and be very painful. Stretching them before the spasms can start can help to keep them limber so that they do not spasm so easily.

My client has lost a lot of muscle mass and so when he relaxes and tries to sleep, the contractions can come from his limbs falling to the side or getting in an awkward position. The movement can increase the pain and so we learned to use extra pillows to prop his legs and arms on and even to keep him from rolling to one side or the other. This helps ease his pain enough that he can take a nap. Because of his pain, he sleeps with several pillows propped all around him.

All of these things I am discussing can be done in conjunction with each other. For example, we have found that massage does well combining it with heat and cold packs. Cold compresses are usually used where there is inflammation such as with a sprained ankle that is red, swollen and inflamed looking. It is also used for inflamed nerves such as back pain and pain down your legs. Sometimes using a cold pack on your face when a really bad headache occurs helps the pain too, especially if it is sinus related.

Heat is excellent for relaxing the muscles that have been strained and soothing them. It is also good for helping strained muscles relax before you start exercising or after you exercise to relax the muscles that have been used during the exercise session. Heat can come in the form of a heat pack or a hot shower, depending on where you hurt and how much area is hurting.

There are massage inserts to put in chairs or to put on the bed that also heat up. That helps a lot of people and it is something a person can do for themselves.

The whole goal of learning alternative methods to use with what your doctor does is to help you go from a victim of chronic illness to a survivor of the pain and then on to a thriver as someone that has learned to find joy in spite of the pain. It is a choice you still have no matter the shape you are in.

Distraction

Distraction means doing something that takes your mind off of the pain and helps divert your attention. There are many forms of distraction and it all depends on what you like to do. It can range from doing things such as getting interested in a movie, listening to music, watching television or other visual things.

There are many ways to use distraction as a form of pain management. I personally like to read as a way to distract myself from chronic pain. I allow my mind to get involved in the story and that takes me away some from the pain. I also lay back in a recliner or on the bed and use pillows to get my body comfortable and then read in a very quiet room. The quietness is soothing.

Other forms of distraction can include knitting, writing, gardening even on a small scale such as potted plants, painting, talking to others. Distraction is anything that takes your mind off the pain. My client loves to sit in the rocking chair and hold the dog and just close his eyes and rub the fur. For him, that is distracting and soothes his pain.

Sometimes distraction can be day dreaming. We all have dreams and aspirations and day dreaming about them is a great distraction. My client loves to day dream about things like tap dancing, or riding a horse. Now he will never do those things again but in his mind, he can race across fields or dance across the stage.

Looking at old pictures and remembering things from the past that are pleasurable is also another form of distraction. Many people love to reminisce about the past and if it is pleasurable, it helps bring some pain relief by the distraction.

The mind is a powerful tool and if we allow pleasurable things to enter our mind and keep the stressful things at bay, it makes the pain easier to bear. Pain can be very isolating and thus very lonely and that increases our pain. My client talks to friends on the computer as a distraction to his pain.

We each have our own things that we like to do or listen to that can be a distraction and so picking which ones is strictly a personal choice.

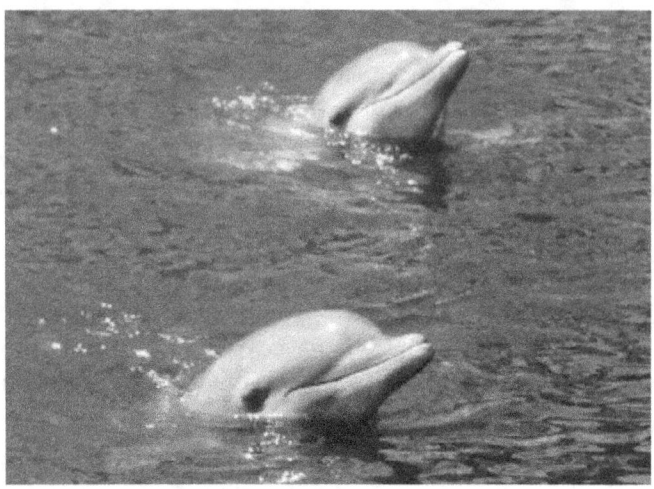

Just keep in mind that dealing with your pain, your chronic illness is all about choice. There are choices out there even when you have lost the ability to do. You can still choose to find joy, choose to do things to help distract yourself, still smile and still enjoy people and those that are joyous in spite of the pain. Those with a good attitude tend to do better with their pain.

My client has a dog and that dog serves as the greatest distraction to him. The dog seems to know when he is feeling the worst and starts doing funny antics as if to make him smile. The affection of the dog is amazing to watch with my client. He will just rub and pet on that dog and hold him as if he were his child and it always seems to soothe him and bring him peace for a while from the pain.

You have choices and so many alternative things and so many things you can use for distraction to help with the pain. When we look to others to entertain us, we will get let down for people are human and have other responsibilities. So, one choice for distraction is learning to pick ones that we can do ourselves.

Visualization

Visualization is a powerful tool to use with pain. It is another term for meditation. I call it meditation with a specific focus. Visualization is guided imagery where you use all of your senses as you visualize the event or behavior that you want. This means, as you visualize, you focus on what you see, what you feel, what you smell, what you hear and incorporate that all into the imagery you are visualizing.

As a person with chronic pain, I use visualization a lot and I visualize that I have army cells that are dressed in warrior armor. I can smell the metal and as I visualize them marching through my veins, I actually allow myself to feel the thump of the marching throughout my body. I visualize that this army surrounds an area of pain and pushes the pain through my veins and out my finger tips.

It took a while to learn how to do this technique but it actually works for me. Other times I visualize I am floating on a river and I can feel the motion of the boat in the water and smell the water and the plants. I can hear the birds. It is all about learning to use your senses and recall things you already know like the sound of birds or running water.

My client and I do a visualization exercise where I talk to him while he is laying on his bed and tell him to visualize that his body has this army inside that is riding great stallions. It is charging up and down his arms and legs rounding up the pain monsters and every time he breathes out, he is blowing the pain monsters out into the ocean.

This is one of those exercises that you really have to be willing to let your imagination work for you. I had a friend who visualized that every time he breathed out he was blowing out cancer cells and he did this daily. No matter what you visualize, let your inner being actually see this inside. Really visualize it. For my friend, he lived ten years with his cancer by using such techniques and he truly believed that it was doing it. He actually blew the breaths into canning jars and sealed the lids because he said he did not want those cells floating out to anyone else.

Create your own visualization and your own army that battles your pain or illness and wins. When you blow out the pain, take deep breaths and blow all the air out and then more until you have no air left before you take another breath so that you are blowing out all the pain each time. Or create a place that you go to when your pain is so bad. Our minds and our bodies are connected and if you can take yourself mentally to another place where there is no pain, it distracts you from the pain at hand.

My client and I both like to use visualization to transport us to a place away from the pain such as the beach or the mountains or flying across the sky. Anything that makes us feel joy. My client visualizes himself dancing and I love when I see him lying on his bed with his eyes closed and his feet are tapping to some inner music. Our minds are powerful and we are only limited by what we allow our minds to feel and see.

When you begin using visualization, and incorporate all your senses, you will find that you can recall certain smells like brownies even though no one is cooking them. All of these things are stored in our brains. Visualization can be used in many forms. Sometimes playing the sound of a waterfall can transport us to a tropical paradise or the scent of jasmine or other flowers or oils can transport us out in nature. All of these things help us to escape the pain for a little while.

Sometimes it helps to have guided visualization to start off. Guided imagery means that someone is leading you through the visualization and telling you what you are seeing. You start off laying down on a coach, bed or recliner and do relaxation type breathing. Then, with eyes closed, make yourself relax by starting with your feet/toes and moving up the legs, fingers and moving up the arms and relaxing the stomach, back, etc and until you are fully relaxed.

When a person is guiding you, have them use all of your senses as they talk gently. As an example, the person may start you off imagining you are resting in a hammock in the back yard where it is quiet and you can smell the scent of fresh mowed grass and you can hear the bees buzzing. This is to help stimulate your senses so that you actually do smell the scent of the grass and hear the bees. There are Guided imagery tapes that you can order if you are alone and want something that guides you through the visualization.

Aroma Therapy

Scents are one of those things that touch a pleasure spot in our brains. Certain foods cooking, certain perfumes, the smell of evergreen transporting us back to the Christmas Holidays, the smell of citrus, chocolate, coffee brewing , tea, cakes cooking, meals cooking, flowers, babies....all of these things can hit a pleasure center that helps transport us away from pain.

Scents can be used with visualization to help transport us even more away from our pain and to a more pleasurable time. And this is just another form of distraction. The smell of Juicy Fruit gum takes me to a memory of my grandmother and I can close my eyes and dream of all the times I remember being with her. And while I am doing that, my brain is not focusing on the pain and so for a while I am transported away from it.

Some places sell aroma therapy items. We have used Lavender oil with my client who finds the smell of it very relaxing and the more he relaxes, the easier his pain becomes. Aroma therapy not only helps with pain but has been shown to help people lower their blood pressure. Some scents are calming and others stimulate and make us want to be more active.

The National Association of Holistic Aromatherapy has a website with a lot of information for people who are interested in aroma therapy. You can locate it at www.naha.org. They even include safety precautions when doing aroma therapy.

Some of the most popular are Lavender which relieves stress, chamomile which is a relaxant, peppermint which is an energizer, rose oil which is supposed to help with anxiety and circulation, rosemary which is supposed to stimulate the brain, and jasmine which is used for its relaxation effect. There are many other aroma therapy oils. Some of these are used in teas also to help in relaxation which in turn will help induce sleep. Always consult your doctor before taking any aroma therapy herb internally so that your doctor can make sure that it will not interfere with the prescription medications that you take.

Certain scents have been found to lessen pain. My belief is that the scents relax us and the more relaxed we are, the less our pain will be. Whether you use candles, oils or herbal teas, these things can help with pain. Again, please consult your doctor before taking anything internally.

Also scents of lotions when doing massage therapy on yourself or someone else has been shown to touch the receptors in our brain that help us relax and feel good. Some people find aroma therapy to not be pleasant to them and you have to decide if scent therapy is for you.

Have you ever noticed how food cooking, especially holiday food brings joyous memories? Sometimes for the man I care for, I will cook pumpkin pie because the scent seems to liven him up and make him want to get up and start moving around the house. It reminds him of his grandmother, who used to cook those pies for him.

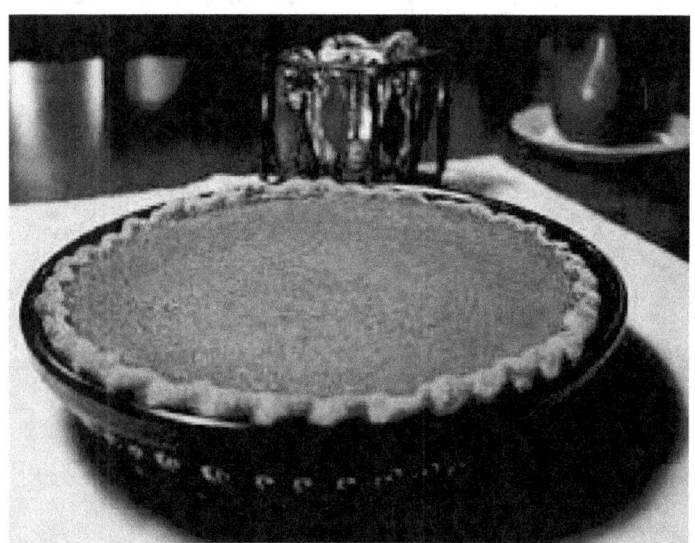

The Power of Music and Dance Therapy

I use music a lot with my client as he loves music. We have learned that music can lift the spirits, lift the heart and energize.

When my client is feeling low because the pain has gnawed at him for hours, he will have me put on music from his era like "Rock Around The Clock" and other songs and he will close his eyes and soon I will see the beginnings of a smile as he becomes totally engulfed in the music and his pain has taken a back seat for a little while.

Sometimes music needs to be soft and soothing like relaxation music and other times, it needs to be music with an upbeat tempo. We use music a lot with visualization for my client loves to dance and so we put on music that he loves and he will lay on the bed or in his chair and close his eyes and visualizes himself dancing around the room. If we allow ourselves to become immersed in the music and the vision, soon we will feel it through our whole body.

Dance therapy is another way to help you transport yourself to another place to escape your pain. Some people, even though they move slowly with chronic pain, are still able to dance. It is amazing to watch the transformation on their faces when the music is playing and they are dancing around the room.

Others can only dance in their chairs but that wonderful mind of theirs transports them to the dance floor. And then others like the man I care for, can only dance when laying on their hospital beds and he closes his eyes and his feet move as he dances around the room in his head.

Dancing as a form of therapy for pain works in conjunction with the distraction suggestion, the power of music suggestion and helps get those natural pain killers in our systems called endorphins moving to help our pain. It is amazing what dancing can do.   And using the hot and cold compress suggestion before and after dancing helps our pain also. If you use the heat on those muscles before you start dancing across the floor, it helps the muscles to relax so that the dancing is so much easier.

Using our imagination and our minds, the world is ours. It is ours to dream and to find methods and daydreams that take us away from the pain and suffering into a better place. Do not be afraid to try and do not feel like it is silly. Nothing is silly if it helps. I had a client once that using one of the new "reborn" dolls that look and feel like a real baby was a diversion from pain technique that worked well. She would sit and rock that baby doll with eyes closed and visualize that she was rocking her own child and you could visibly see the pain leave her face.

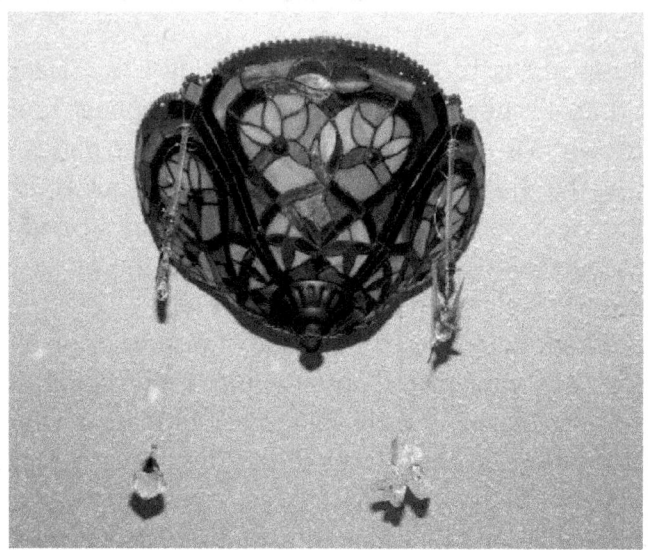

So, allow yourself to be free and to expand your senses and your mind to incorporate what children have done for years. Children are quick healers because they do not hold on to the negative or the pain like we adults tend to do.

Create diversion things in your space like the stained glass ceiling light with glass mobiles of hummingbirds and flowers hanging from it. It is a wonderful visualization device for someone laying on their bed and needing to escape the pain.

Using Assistive Devices

I have discovered that many people make their lives harder because they refuse to use assistive devices or assistive methods. I believe they associate them with being old and so will not use them. Unfortunately, when you need an assistive device such as a cane, walker, raised toilet seat, grab bars, ramps, and even moving things closer to your chair such as your computer so that you can sit in a softer chair rather than a desk chair and you refuse to use them, you only increase your pain and raise your risk of falling.

My client spends most of his time in a hospital bed or in his recliner due to the pain. So, we fixed a table by his bed so that his monitor to his computer sits on it and he can put the keyboard on a tray in his lap when he is propped up in bed. This way he can type in bed and see his monitor beside him. Or he can sit in his recliner and put a pillow in his lap and type and see his monitor which sits on a table beside his chair. This gives him such a great deal of pleasure because he socializes on the computer. And if we had not done this, he would not be able to use the computer at all.

Assistive devices are just what the name says. They are things to assist you in daily living. They are designed to make life easier and thereby lessen the pain of trying to do it on your own. When you refuse to use them, you are making your life harder and you are making it harder on those who love you and take care of you.

My grandparents refused to use their walkers and other devices and both of them made it so hard for my mother and her siblings all because of the danger of their falls and because not using the walker meant that my grandparents could not take care of themselves.

I have had clients that refused to use walkers and ended up falling. I have had other ones tell me that they were not going to move things around to make it easier and would say they were not that old yet. And yet, all they did was deprive themselves from doing things.

Assistive devices can include a hospital bed, a gel mattress or memory foam mattress to make the bed more comfortable. It can also include using larger ink pens, big handled silverware, special devices that help you put your shoes and socks on or help you wash your feet and back in the shower.

They can also include things like a TENS unit which stimulate the nerves to help by pass the pain such as in back pain. I use a TENS unit to help on those days when my back pain is really high and the electrical stimulation actually distracts me from the actual pain.

Many people do not try the TENS unit because it does not totally remove the pain. We have to keep in mind that there will always be some pain. It is the high pain we are trying to help lower.

Sometimes you can make modifications to very simple things that keep you from increasing your pain. For example, the small knobs on lamps can be replaced with a pull chain. Using a pump bottle for lotions and shampoos, etc is much easier than using the kind that you have to squeeze which can hurt arthritic hands.

Another assistive device is biofeedback. It helps you to recognize your own behavior and those things that are increasing your pain and those that lessen your pain. Personal biofeedback machines can be bought for about seventy dollars and it lets you know when you are doing things that are increasing you pain.

I have learned to recognize in myself when I am doing things that make my pain worse and there by learn to avoid or to take immediate measures to try to keep the pain from going higher. Biofeedback is a way of teaching you to relax naturally which helps to decrease your pain. Learning when to recognize that you are stressed or allowing anxiety to grow and then learning how to stop what you are doing that is causing this is what biofeedback is all about.

I personally find that keeping a journal helps. When my pain starts rising, I make a note of what I was doing, what was going on and what I did for the pain. After days of doing this, I was able to look back and see that at certain times of day my anxiety from pain rose and that by eating a small snack and resting, my pain was lowered greatly.

Other ways to assist in helping your pain is by being aware of your surroundings and what you do. For example, keep a smaller pocketbook for the weight can increase pain when you have to carry it very far. Quit throwing your bag over your shoulder for the extra weight on one shoulder can cause pain.

Going to the grocery story is hard for people with chronic pain and so learning to use the store scooters, having a small dolly type thing to carry your bags to the car and into the house, making sure that they do not overload your bags at the checkout counter so that you are not carrying too heavy a bag is essential in making the shopping less painful.

If you live in a house with stairs, keep duplicate things on each floor like your hairbrush, toothbrush, change of clothing, etc so that you do not have to run up and down the stairs all day getting these things. Get assistive things for the kitchen such as electric can openers, jar openers, etc. All of these things are ways to assist yourself and help keep from increasing your pain.

It is all about making life easier and maintaining independence. The longer a person can remain independent, the healthier they are emotionally for no one really wants to be dependent on someone else. But, it takes those with health problems being willing to try assistive devices and to try alternative methods.

I had a client that I will call Bob who became severely depressed when he could not move around like he used to. He shut himself off to the world and the only people that he allowed in were the caretakers. He did not even want his family there and they were missing him greatly. It took a very small grandchild to make him realize that he was depriving everyone else and himself.

When the small child asked Bob why he did not let them visit anymore, Bob told him it was because his legs no longer worked and that he could not do anything. The little boy looked at his grandfather and said simply "but I didn't come to see your legs grandpa".

Watching from a distance, I could see that those words struck a chord in Bob and he soon started opening himself up to the wheelchair and to allowing the family back in. It is all a choice and we have to choose wisely for we can never regain time.

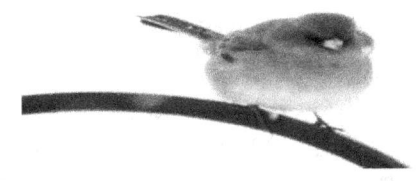

Support therapy

I saved this one for last because I think it is so important. Often, people in chronic pain are alone a big percentage of the time. And having someone to talk to about the pain is very important. The support groups on the internet have helped many people because there are people there that are going through what you are going through.

Feeling alone and isolated because of chronic pain can increases your pain because it creates a stress within you and stress makes pain worse. Getting out and being around other people is a way to help the loneliness. Many people cannot tolerate being around crowds of people but just one person to talk to can help.

If you cannot get out, the internet has so many options. There is Skype that allows you to see the person you are talking to and makes you feel like the person is right there with you. My client uses Skype to talk to family and loved ones so that he does not feel alone all the time. If you have never used Skype, there are messenger programs online that allow you to talk to people in real time by typing to them. We all need that connection with others. It helps us to cope with chronic pain and it also can help distract us from it when we talk to those we love.

The American Chronic Pain Association has a link that allows you to put in your state and find where chronic pain support groups are in your area. The link is located here:

http://www.theacpa.org/33/SupportGroups.aspx

Also, if you put "chronic pain" in your search engine, there are numerous sites that have support groups that have people who suffer with chronic pain as members. Support is vital in dealing with chronic pain.

Opening our minds and allowing our creative energies to help us with pain is nothing new. It has been going on for years. Some people are afraid to let themselves try it. Others want the ease of just having more pain medicine. But, those that do try alternative ways to deal with pain have found that not only does it help with chronic pain but it also enhances their life by giving them things they had not been able to do for a long time.

Thoughts for the Person who has a loved one that lives with Chronic Pain

- Being around someone in chronic pain is not always easy. People who suffer with chronic pain are fighting a battle that can make them hard to deal with not because they are a bad patient but because they are fighting with all they have to deal with the chronic pain.

- Often their world narrows as they lose interest in other things including you. They do not mean to but dealing with too many things when you are fighting chronic pain sometimes becomes impossible.

- Never tell them you know exactly how they feel for unless you deal with chronic pain day in and day out; you do not know how they feel. A back ache or a headache will go away. There is an ending to it. With chronic pain, there is no ending for most people. Can you imagine that? Knowing that your backache or headache or toothache will never end? That is what a person with chronic pain deals with.

- Do not tell them to take their medicine and it will be better because it most likely will not be better. Pain meds do not remove all the pain. The hope is that they will help control the pain for a chronic pain user.

- Try to make accommodations for those with chronic pain. No, they cannot do all the things they used to do but if people are willing to bend a little, they can still be involved. Make sure there is some where comfortable for the person with chronic pain or somewhere to lie down if they get tired.

- Please do not tell them to just take another pain pill and "let's go". It does not work that way.

- Please be kind and gentle with your loved ones with chronic pain. It is already a painful journey and they do not need emotional pain on top of it from people who do not understand what chronic pain is.

- A person with chronic pain just wants you to be there and to love them. They do not expect you to bring cures or to fix it. Sometimes they are content to just sit in silence knowing you are right there with them.

- A person with chronic pain has already lost part of their lives to the pain; please do not abandon them because it takes more time to have them be with you. I see so many who are alone and no family or friends come to visit.

- Most importantly, just love them. That is the greatest thing you can give them. Love them and do things to make life a little easier such as bringing meals to them or helping them in cleaning their house or their yard. Most will never ask for help but if you offer, they most likely will not turn it down.

- The patient I take care of has a great sense of humor but I can tell you that he does not like you to make jokes when he is trying to talk seriously about his health to you. He says it is demeaning.

- Living with chronic pain does not mean a person has lost their intellect. It means they are fighting pain. It does not mean they have lost their hearing. They are fighting pain. It does not mean they do not want to be involved. They just need some special concessions that really do not take that much time.

- Try to learn the pain schedule of someone dealing with chronic pain. For example, my client's pain is worse in the afternoons, so if family or friends want to do things with him, they need to schedule it in the mornings.

- Most of all be an advocate for your loved one in pain not an adversary.

ABOUT THE AUTHORS

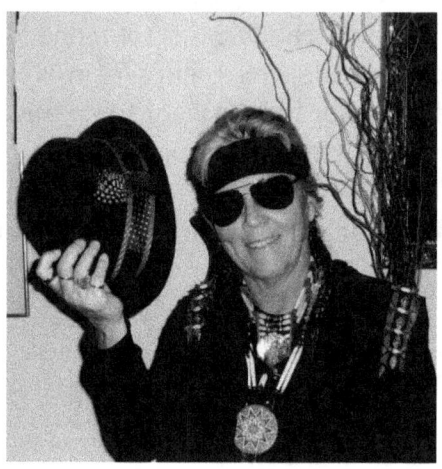

Sherry E. Showalter, Ph.D., L.C.S.W. is a **National Heart of Hospice** recipient for psycho-social-spiritual care-giving. Dr. Showalter has been a long time advocate for patients and families coping with pain, chronic pain, loss, dying and bereavement. She proudly served with other first responders at the Pentagon during 9/11 and continues to work with those coping with chronic pain and sudden and traumatic loss. She is a keynote speaker and psychotherapist. Dr. Showalter is Native American and believes in many alternative methods to help with chronic pain. She is also the author of **Healing Heartaches: Stories of Loss and Life** and **Down The Hallway.**

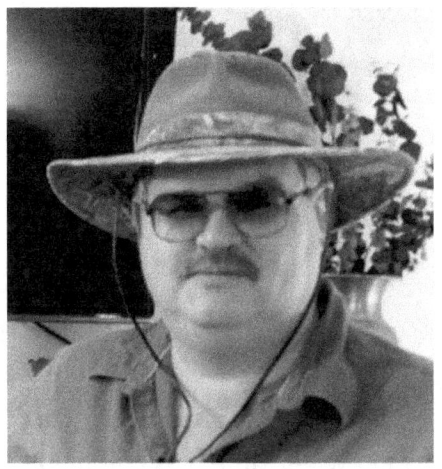

John Argent is a full time caretaker and deals with those living with chronic pain and has dealt with his own chronic pain. He worked in emergency management and 911 for 12 years, was a volunteer firefighter and is a certified First Responder. Through the years, he has learned many alternative ways to deal with chronic pain and to help those that he takes care of enhance the methods their physicians use. He is currently working on two novels he hopes to complete in the near future; **Evil Comes To Town** and **From Son To Caretaker.**

The Last Dance

With wisps of hair across her beautiful face

Tears on her cheeks your finger could trace

She stood there with head bowed in humble prayer

Feeling as if she were the only one that cared

She closed her eyes and listened once more

To the music that always drew her to the door

The music rose in tempo and sound

She knew her time was coming around

Was her dream to dance just one last dance

And she knew tonight was her only chance

Rising on toes, she danced across the stage

Her body tensing up for the very next page

As she jumped to twirl up in the air

She suddenly felt his hands right there

He lifted her higher than she had ever flown

And twirled and danced better than she had ever known

He molded himself to her as if one

And remained there lifting her until the dance was done

The applause thundered and echoed around the room

And she felt as if life had just started to bloom

As the sounds died down, she smiled with tears

Not being able to dance was one of her fears

Then she opened her eyes and looked around

Oxygen hoses and hospital beds are what she found

As she glanced down she saw her toes pointed down

And she knew only her attitude kept her bed bound

No matter what happened she could dance so free

She just had to close her eyes and the stage she would see

danLrene 2013

Never give up. Use what you have to make life as beautiful as you can and when you no longer can do something, use your mind to do it.

www.ingramcontent.com/pod-product-compliance
Lightning Source LLC
Chambersburg PA
CBHW072342290526
45794CB00002B/986